SOCIAL EMOTIONAL LEARNING (SEL)

Student Planner Grades K-2

Title: Social Emotional Learning (SEL) Student Planner Grades K-2

ISBN: 978-1-7336417-0-8

Authors:
Rebecca Criollo
Hyam Elsaharty
Jennifer N. Laster
Laura Richard
Michelle M. Torres

Editors:
Janna Nobleza
Elisa Flammini

Published 2020 by Seltrove, an imprint of Edtrove
Copyright Edtrove Ltd. and IB Source, Inc.

Table of Contents

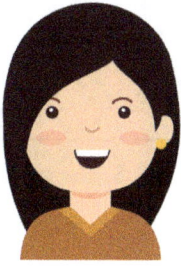 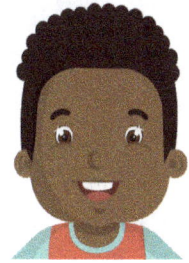

Who am I?

My name: _____

My address:

_____

_____

My Class information:

Teacher: _____

Grade: _____

Room number: _____

School year: _____

Emergency Contact Information:

Name:

_____

Relationship to Student: _____

Telephone: _____

Email: _____

Name:

_____

Relationship to Student: _____

Telephone: _____

Email: _____

Known Allergies:

_____

_____

My favorites:

Color: _____

Animal: _____

Book: _____

Movie: _____

Song: _____

Food: _____

Hobby: _____

Sport: _____

I'm special because _____

_____

_____

_____

_____

_____

_____

_____

This year, I'm most looking forward to

_____

_____

_____

_____

_____

_____

_____

_____

_____

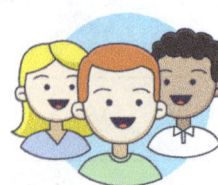

Draw a picture of yourself

My Planner

Hi! This planner is for you! It is a place for you to write your homework. It is also a place for you to learn and practice your SEL skills. Throughout this planner you will learn how to:

- Recognize your emotions and develop confidence. (Self-Awareness)
- Create and maintain friendships and communicate with others. (Relationships Skills)
- Respect other people and empathize with others. (Social Awareness)
- Set goals for yourself and feel calm. (Self-Management)
- Solve problems and reflect. (Responsible Descision-Making)

In this planner, you will:

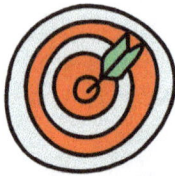

Set goals on the **Goals** pages, check in on your goals throughout the year, and then reflect on your goals at the end of this planner.

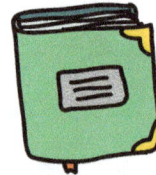

Explore each of the skills above in the **Theme** pages with books to read and activities to do so you can learn about each theme.

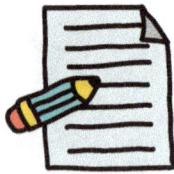

Review each skill at the end of the theme.

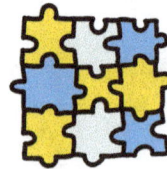

Make **connections** between each skill and books you have read at school or at home.

At the end of this planner, you will find pages to help you continue learning about your SEL skills.

- A Dictionary of Emotions to help you know how you feel and what you can do about your feelings.

- Ways to be mindful and calm.

- What to say when you are having a disagreement with someone.

- A class activity so your whole class can work together well.

- Stories of students just like you who solved their problems using their SEL skills.

- How to use SEL in your life.

- Things you can say to yourself to make yourself feel confident and happier.

You can share what you are learning with your parents or carer at home, too. The adults in your life want you to feel good about yourself, learn more about how your brain and heart respond to things, and have friends who you can rely on!

As you use this planner, if there is something you don't understand, ask a trusted adult. They can help you!

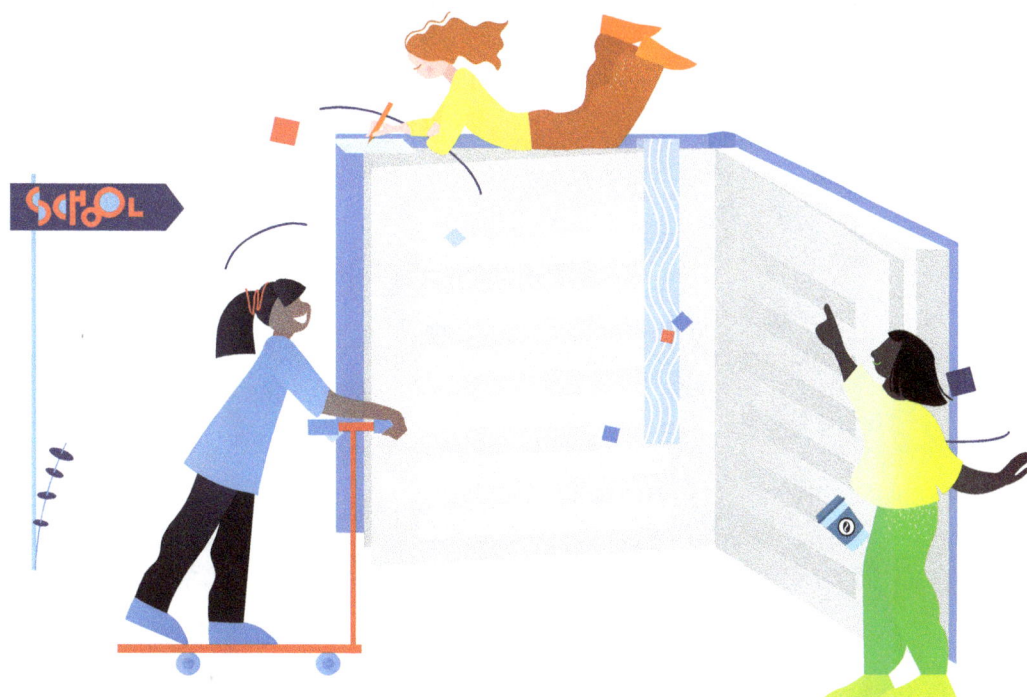

Notes

Notes

Goals

A goal is something that you want to be able to do, learn, or accomplish. Sometimes, we set goals that we want to achieve over a long amount of time, and other times, we set goals that we want to achieve in a shorter amount of time. Usually, we have some of both types of goals at the same time.

When we make goals, we want them to be things we can achieve, so if something seems really big, think about how you can break it down into smaller goals. For example, instead of saying that you want to be a famous singer, you might break it down and say that you need to learn how to sing, so you will take voice lessons. Also, you need to make sure the goals you set are specific and something that you can measure or track. For example, if you just say get better at something, what does that mean? How will you know when you are better at it? Think of what you mean when you say you want to get better at it and write that instead. When you set a goal, make sure it is something that you can control. For example, don't set a goal that there will be 100 sunny days this school year. That is not something that you can control or work towards.

One of the most important things about goals is to celebrate your successes. You can celebrate when you've accomplished one of the steps that will help you to reach your goal and when you achieve your goal, too!

Goals for this year

To write a goal, you need to include what you want to achieve, and by when you will achieve it. You could use the following sentence frame, or something similar: "I want to _____ by _____."

Write 3 goals for this school year. Try to include different types of goals: academic (learning), social (friends/family), activities (dance, sports, music, play, etc.), or others.

Goal 1

Goal #1: _____

_____

_____

_____

_____

Date you will accomplish this goal: _____

Steps you will take to reach this goal:

1. _____

_____

2. _____

_____

3. _____

_____

Who can you ask for help with this goal? _____

How will you know you've accomplished this goal? _____

_____

_____

_____

_____

_____

Goal 2

Goal #2: _____

_____

_____

_____

_____

Date you will accomplish this goal: _____

Steps you will take to reach this goal:

1. _____

_____

2. _____

_____

3. _____

_____

Who can you ask for help with this goal? _____

How will you know you've accomplished this goal? _____

_____

_____

_____

_____

Goal 3

Goal #3: _____

_____

_____

_____

_____

Date you will accomplish this goal: _____

Steps you will take to reach this goal:

1. _____

_____

2. _____

_____

3. _____

_____

Who can you ask for help with this goal? _____

How will you know you've accomplished this goal? _____

_____

_____

_____

_____

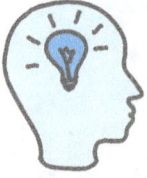

Identity and Mindset

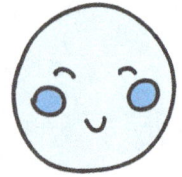

The next 10 weeks will focus on identity and mindset with an emphasis on the social-emotional competency of self-awareness.

You will practice:
1. What emotion am I feeling when I feel a certain way? (Identifying emotions)
2. What does this emotion feel like in my body? (Identifying emotions)
3. What am I good at? (Recognizing strengths / Self-confidence)
4. How can I be a good friend to my classmates? (Accurate self-perception)
5. How can I solve problems by myself or ask for help to solve them? (Self-efficacy)

You and your carer can learn more about identity and mindset by reading books together at home. Here are some good books that focus on the topic of identity and mindset (and remember you don't have to buy the book to read it; you can check the books out at your school or community's library):

Recognizing Strengths / Self-confidence / Self-perception / Self-efficacy

The Dot by Peter H. Reynolds
The Best Kind of Bear by Greg Gormley
Hair Love by Matthew A. Cherry
Sulwe by Lupita Nyong'o
Eraser by Anna Kang
Counting on Katherine by Helaine Becker

Identifying emotions

The Feeling Flower by Lea Mahealani Dakroub
When Sophie gets Angry -- Really, Really Angry by Molly Bang
Me and My Fear by Francesca Sanna
When Sadness is at your Door by Eva Eland
The Color Monster by Anna Llenas
The Heart and the Bottle by Oliver Jeffers

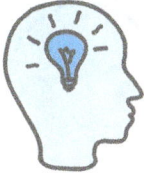

Identity and Mindset

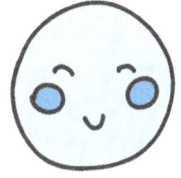

Everyone has things that define who they are as people. Some of these things are similar to ours, whereas others are different. We can see some of these things, but then there are other things that we cannot see. In this game, you need to stand up and walk around the room meeting your classmates. Find a different person for each description below. Write the name of your new friend on the line of the description matching that person. You need to find a different person for each of the 16 boxes below.

Find Someone Who...

Has two siblings. _____	Loves roller coasters. _____	Wears socks to bed. _____	Has been on an airplane. _____
Has brown eyes. _____	Has a pet. _____	Likes very spicy food. _____	Wears glasses. _____
Loves to swim. _____	Likes to play soccer. _____	Takes dance class. _____	Has painted fingernails. _____
Has been camping. _____	Likes to read. _____	Sings in the shower. _____	Likes creating art. _____

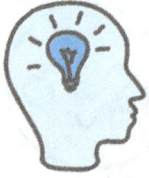

All About Me

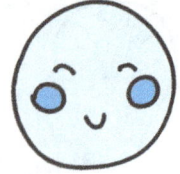

Every person is unique and special. Think about all the things that make you unique: your name, your family, your likes and favorites, your personality, your beliefs, your culture, and a lot more. All these things make you special. Over time, some of these things will stay the same, while others will change.

Practice:

In the space below, decorate the figure to show who you are. Make it look like you and surround it with people and/or things that are important to you.

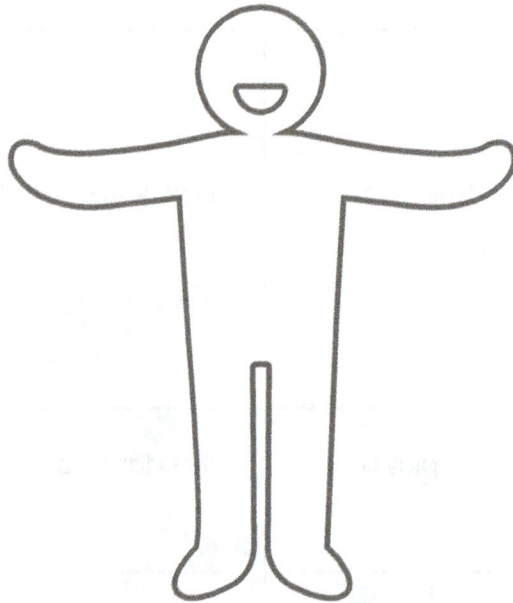

Extension:

Look at your figure and decide what things may stay the same and what may change about who you are over time. Talk with a partner about what you notice.

Learning Log

My goal this week: _____

_____

		Minutes Read:
Monday	_____ _____ _____ _____	_____
Tuesday	_____ _____ _____ _____	Minutes Read: _____
Wednesday	_____ _____ _____ _____	Minutes Read: _____
Thursday	_____ _____ _____ _____	Minutes Read: _____
Friday	_____ _____ _____ _____	Minutes Read: _____
Home/School Communication		

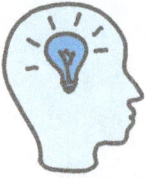

Making Friends

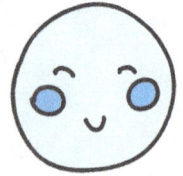

According to the dictionary, a friend is "a person who you like and enjoy being with." At home, you live with your family, but at school, you are surrounded by classmates, who then become your friends. The first thing you need to do to make a friend is introduce yourself to them. Next, you can talk about the things that you like, for example: games, toys, and books that you enjoy. You can also find something that you both enjoy doing together. The important thing to remember about friends is that they have feelings, just like you, so please think about how your actions affect them.

Practice:
Make a comic strip showing two people who are about to become friends. Try to draw what they do and write what they say and how they feel.

Extension:
Use puppets to act out how two people who are becoming friends talk to each other. What do the puppets say to each other? How do they behave toward each other? What do they do that shows you they are becoming friends?

Learning Log

My goal this week: _____

_____

		Minutes Read:
Monday	_____ _____ _____ _____	_____
Tuesday	_____ _____ _____ _____	_____
Wednesday	_____ _____ _____ _____	_____
Thursday	_____ _____ _____ _____	_____
Friday	_____ _____ _____ _____	_____
Home/School Communication		

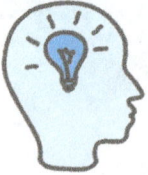

Asking to Play

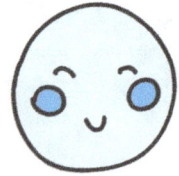

Sometimes, you see a group of kids playing and you want to play with them, too. Usually, all you need to do is to ask to play in order to join the game they're playing. Try asking if you can join them. Sometimes, it is more effective to suggest a specific way that you can add to the play. For example, if you see a few kids playing school, you could ask if you could be the music teacher. The other kids might suggest a different role for you to play. You can then decide if you'd like to play that role or if you'd like to do something else. There may be times when what you'd like to play doesn't work with the game that is already being played, so you and the other kids will have to decide the things that you can do together within that game.

Practice:

Haanan and D'Angelo are playing restaurant in the play kitchen. Edison sees them playing and wants to join them. What should he do?

_____

_____

At recess, a group of kids are playing Superheroes. Josefina wants to play with them, too. What should she do?

_____

_____

A group of kids are playing hospital. Keiko goes over to the group and tells them that she wants to play and that she wants to be the doctor. They tell her that she can't be the doctor because they already have a doctor in the game they're playing. What should she do next?

_____

_____

Extension:

In small groups, role play scenarios in which someone wants to play with other kids. What types of words are best when asking to join in play? How does the way that you ask to play depend on the situation?

Learning Log

My goal this week: _____

_____

		Minutes Read:
Monday	_____ _____ _____ _____	_____
Tuesday	_____ _____ _____ _____	_____
Wednesday	_____ _____ _____ _____	_____
Thursday	_____ _____ _____ _____	_____
Friday	_____ _____ _____ _____	_____
Home/School Communication		

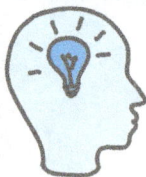

Personal space

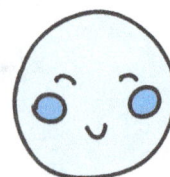

Everyone has a body and around their body, they have personal space. Personal space is the space that is right around your body. Some people like to have a lot of personal space around them without other people too close to them. Other people don't mind having less personal space, or even being touched by others. When sharing space in a classroom, it is important to notice where other people's bodies are and try to respect their personal space by not moving our own bodies into it. These are some important rules about personal space:

1. Pay attention to how close your body is to the personal space of other people.
2. Pay attention to how other people react when you are close to them or touch them.
3. If someone is in your personal space and you don't like it, use your words to tell them how you feel. You could say, "I don't like it when you're in my personal space, please back up." or "I feel uncomfortable when you're in my personal space, please back up."

Practice:

One way to think about personal space is to imagine a space bubble, which is like a giant invisible balloon. Use your imagination to take your space bubble out. Now, blow it up until it is big enough to fit around your whole body. Put it around your body. This is your personal space. You should not get into other people's space bubbles and they should not get into yours.

Sometimes, the size of your space bubble changes depending on who you're with.

Draw yourself in your space bubble when you're with your family:

Draw yourself in your space bubble when you're with people you don't know, like at the store:

What would you say to someone if they came into your personal space and you didn't like it?

_____

_____

Extension:
Play a game with your friends where you are all in space bubbles. Try not to touch each other at all as you walk around the room! Is it easy or difficult to stay out of people's space bubbles?

Learning Log

My goal this week: _____

_____

		Minutes Read:
Monday	_____ _____ _____ _____	_____
Tuesday	_____ _____ _____ _____	Minutes Read: _____
Wednesday	_____ _____ _____ _____	Minutes Read: _____
Thursday	_____ _____ _____ _____	Minutes Read: _____
Friday	_____ _____ _____ _____	Minutes Read: _____
Home/School Communication		

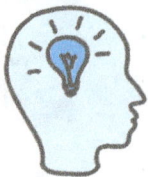 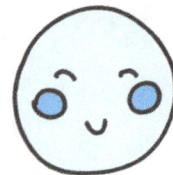

Identifying Emotions

Emotions is another word for feelings. We all can have different kinds of emotions. There are no good or bad feelings; there are just feelings. It is important to find out how we are feeling, so that we know the best way to deal with those emotions. It can also be helpful to learn to figure out other people's emotions so that we can respond to them in the proper way.

To identify our emotions, we need to think about how we are feeling inside and how we are reacting to what is happening around us. To figure out other people's emotions, we need to look at a person's face and body language. What do these things tell us? We use this information to decide how we, or someone else, is feeling.

Practice:
Draw what a person's face looks like when they feel the emotions written below. Make sure you include as many details as possible.

Happy

Sad

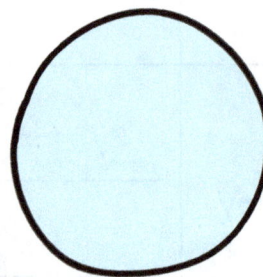

Angry

Scared

Extension:
With a partner, take turns showing emotions with your face and body. Then, have the other person guess which emotion you're showing. Which emotion is the easiest to guess? Which emotion is more difficult to guess? Why do you think that is?

Learning Log

My goal this week: _____

_____

		Minutes Read:
Monday	_____ _____ _____ _____	_____
Tuesday	_____ _____ _____ _____	Minutes Read: _____
Wednesday	_____ _____ _____ _____	Minutes Read: _____
Thursday	_____ _____ _____ _____	Minutes Read: _____
Friday	_____ _____ _____ _____	Minutes Read: _____
Home/School Communication		

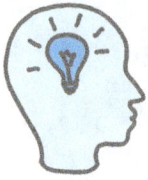

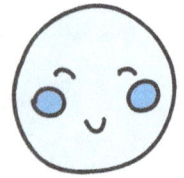

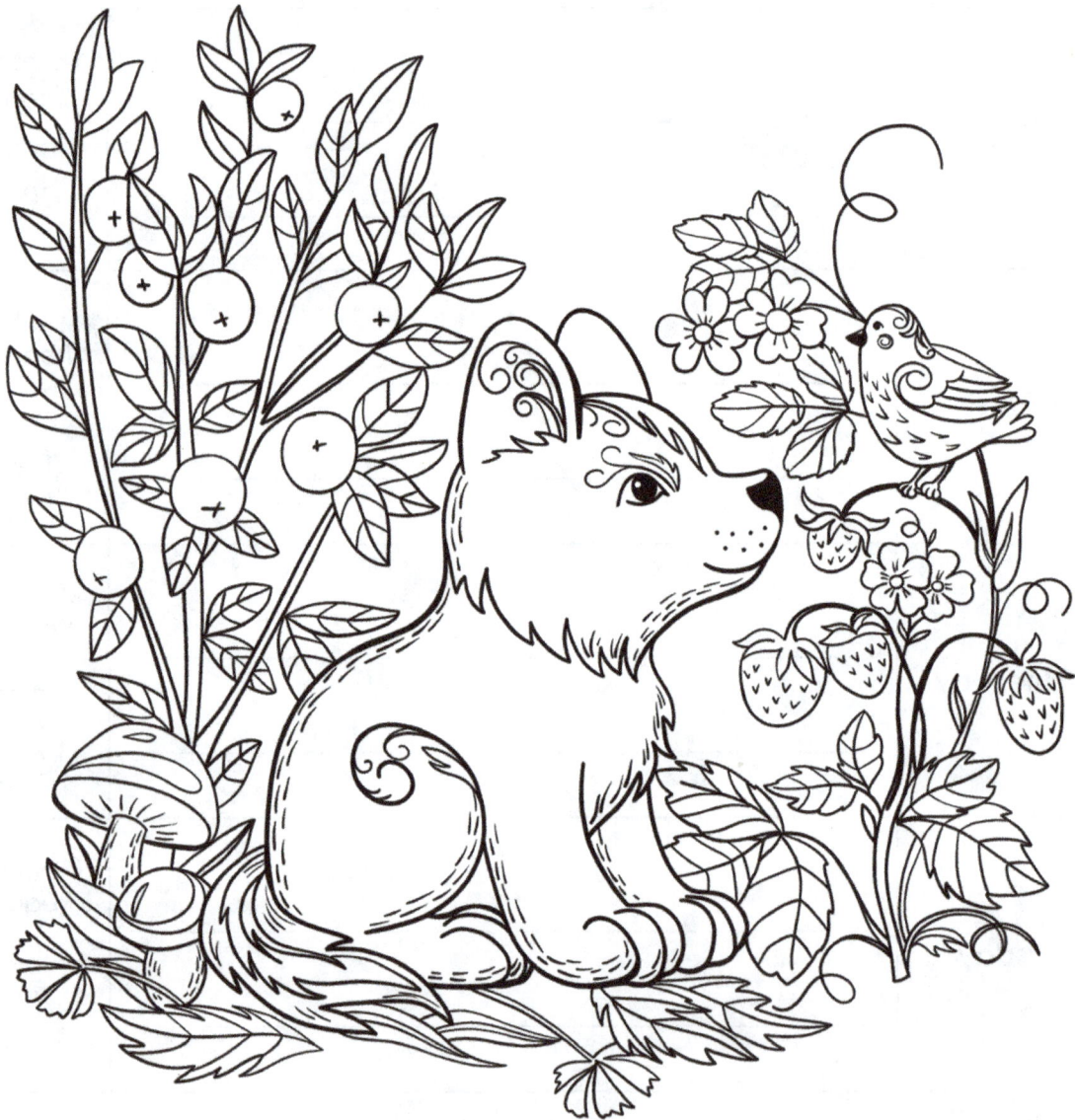

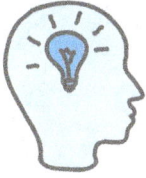

COLORING PAGE

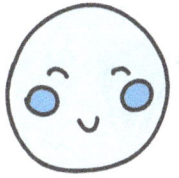

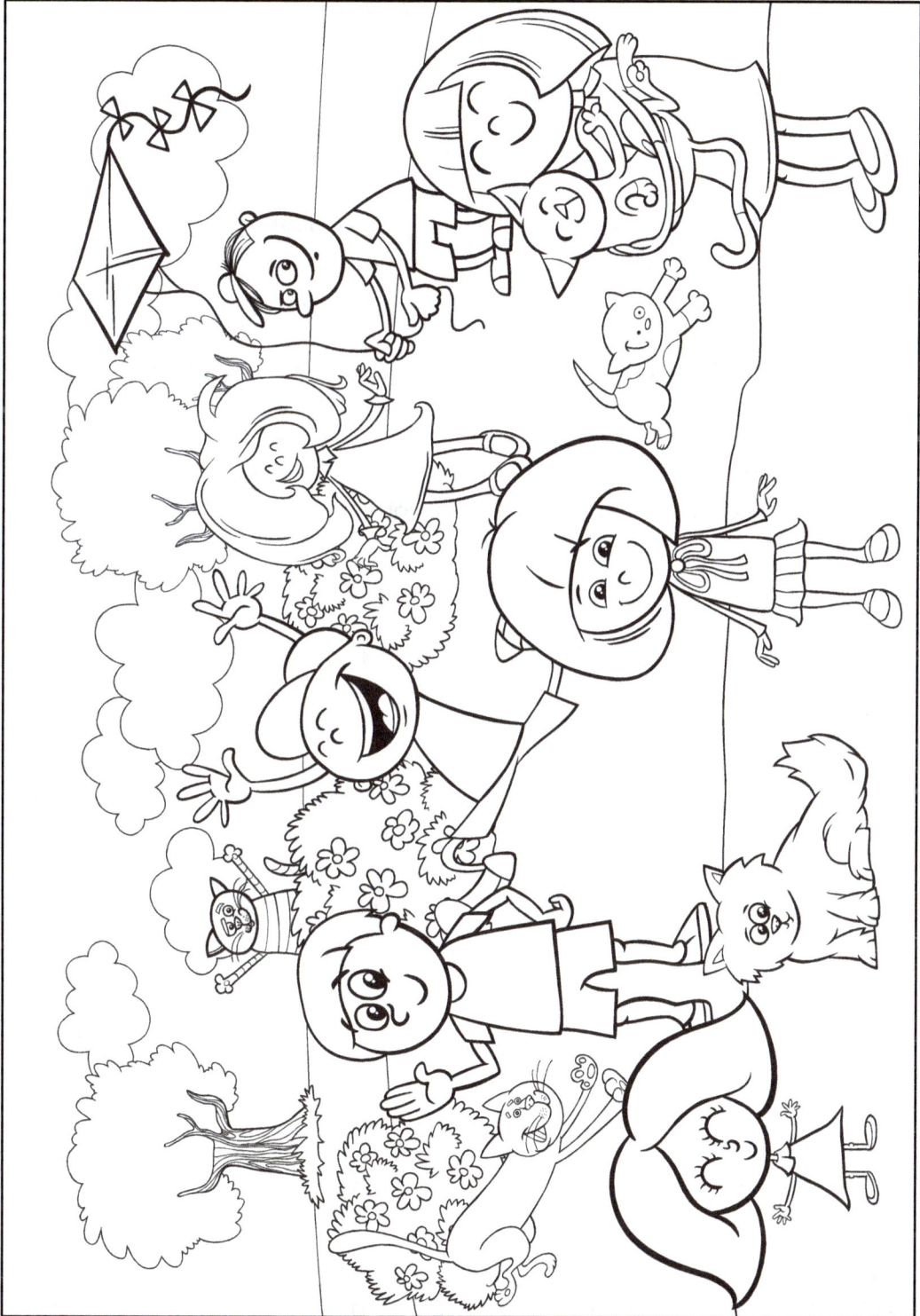

COLORING PAGE

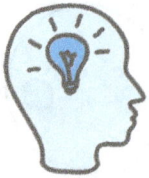

Emotions I:
Angry, Frustrated, Jealous

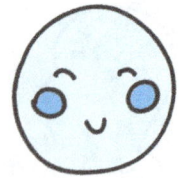

Emotions are not good or bad. It is helpful to notice how you and others are feeling in order to respond in a proper way. It is important to say how you're feeling so that other people can understand.

Angry = When you feel mad.
What to do: First, take a deep breath or take a minute to be quiet or calm. When you feel calmer, you can explain how you are feeling, what is making you feel that way, and look for a solution. Some things you can do when you are feeling angry include: drawing, writing, moving your body (running, playing a sport, etc.), spending some time by yourself, and meditation.

Frustrated = When you feel angry or unhappy because you are trying to do something, but are not being successful.
What to do: First, take a break from what you are doing. Try taking a deep breath or taking a minute to be quiet and think about the best thing to do next. When you feel calmer, it becomes easier to explain to someone else what you are trying to do and ask for help.

Jealous = When you feel unhappy or angry because someone else has something that you want or is doing something that you want to do.
What to do: Talk to someone about how you are feeling. Think about the people and things in your life that you are grateful for. If there is a way to change the situation you are feeling jealous about, work towards making that change.

Practice:
Reflect on a time when you felt one of these emotions.

	Emotion (circle one): Angry Frustrated Jealous
What happened?	
What did you do?	

Extension:
Write and illustrate a story about a kid who felt one of these emotions. You could use *When Sophie Gets Angry—Really, Really Angry* by Molly Bang as a model for your story.

Learning Log

My goal this week: _____

_____

		Minutes Read:
Monday	_____ _____ _____ _____	_____
Tuesday	_____ _____ _____ _____	Minutes Read: _____
Wednesday	_____ _____ _____ _____	Minutes Read: _____
Thursday	_____ _____ _____ _____	Minutes Read: _____
Friday	_____ _____ _____ _____	Minutes Read: _____
Home/School Communication		

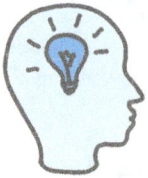

Emotions 2:
Scared, Nervous, Sad, Disappointed

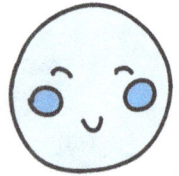

Emotions are not good or bad. It can be helpful to notice how you and others are feeling so that you can respond appropriately. It is important to clearly say how you're feeling so that other people can understand.

Scared = When you feel afraid.
What to do: Talk to someone about why you are scared. Try taking small steps toward doing things that you feel scared of with someone you trust.

Nervous = When you feel worried or are afraid of what might happen.
What to do: Tell someone how you are feeling, so that they can understand and try to help. Talk to them about what might happen. Ask questions. Make a plan for what you can do. When you feel nervous, it is helpful to take deep breaths in order to feel calmer.

Sad = When you feel unhappy.
What to do: Talk to someone about how you feel. It's OK to cry. Spend time with people who make you feel safe and find things you enjoy doing.

Disappointed = When you feel unhappy because something you hoped for did not happen.
What to do: Tell someone how you are feeling. Think about what you could do to make things better. Is there anything good that can come from this situation?

Practice:
Choose one of the emotions above that you've experienced before. Draw a before and after picture of what happened and what you did about it. Add writing if you want to.

Emotion: _____

Before	**After**

Extension:
Make something you could use to help you when you're feeling one of these emotions. It could be a card that reminds you what you can do, something to hold when you're nervous, or a picture to cheer you up when you're feeling sad. Where will you keep this so that you can find it when you need it?

Learning Log

My goal this week: _____

_____

		Minutes Read:
Monday	_____ _____ _____ _____	_____
Tuesday	_____ _____ _____ _____	Minutes Read: _____
Wednesday	_____ _____ _____ _____	Minutes Read: _____
Thursday	_____ _____ _____ _____	Minutes Read: _____
Friday	_____ _____ _____ _____	Minutes Read: _____
Home/School Communication		

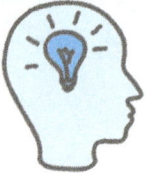

Emotions 3:
Happy, Confident, Proud, Excited

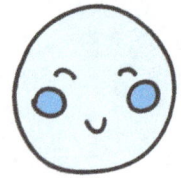

Emotions are not good or bad. It is helpful to notice how you and others are feeling in order to respond appropriately. It's important to say how you're feeling so other people can understand.

Happy = When you feel joy.
What to do: Enjoy this feeling. Try to share your happiness with others by playing with them, sharing with them, or being extra kind.

Confident = When you believe you can do something well.
What to do: Remember how being confident feels in your body because there will be times when you do something and don't feel confident. Consider how you could build confidence when you are working on or doing something where you don't feel confident.

Proud = When you feel happy because you did something well.
What to do: Congratulate yourself for a job well done. Share your pride with a carer like your mom or a teacher; they will be proud of you! When you feel pride, be careful not to put down others who may not find it as easy to do.

Excited = When you feel excited or enthusiastic.
What to do: Laugh, smile, and share your excitement with others. Sometimes when we feel excited we are in a place where we need to be calm or quiet, though, and this can be hard since excited can be a louder emotion. If you need to, calm your body by breathing deeply.

Practice:
Choose one of the above emotions. Write about a time when you felt that emotion. What made you feel that way? What did you do?

_____

_____

_____

Extension:
Now that you've learned about a lot of different emotions, sing a version of "If You're Happy and You Know It." As a class, decide on which emotion words and movements/sounds you'll make for each emotion we have covered throughout these past three weeks after the first verse. Was it harder to come up with movements/sounds for some emotions than others? Why do you think that is?

Learning Log

My goal this week: _____

_____

		Minutes Read:
Monday	_____ _____ _____ _____	Minutes Read: _____
Tuesday	_____ _____ _____ _____	Minutes Read: _____
Wednesday	_____ _____ _____ _____	Minutes Read: _____
Thursday	_____ _____ _____ _____	Minutes Read: _____
Friday	_____ _____ _____ _____	Minutes Read: _____
Home/School Communication		

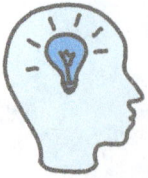

Self-Talk

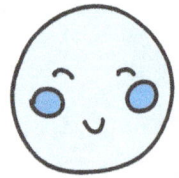

Self-talk is what we say to ourselves, usually quietly in our heads, but sometimes even aloud. We can use self-talk to encourage ourselves to do our best when we are working on something, like writing, or drawing. We can use self-talk to motivate us to try doing something that might seem hard to do. When we use positive self-talk, it can help make us feel more confident and achieve success. A couple simple ways to use positive self-talk is to tell yourself, "I can do this" or "I can succeed."

Sometimes, our self-talk can be negative and it is important that we notice when we are saying negative things to ourselves. When we notice that our self-talk is negative and we are saying things like, "I can't..." we need to turn it around and start using positive self-talk instead.

Practice:

What are three situations in which you could use self-talk? (Example: Trying a new food.)

1. _____

2. _____

3. _____

What would you say to yourself in each of those situations? (Example: I might like this food.)

1. _____

2. _____

3. _____

Extension:

As a class, make a class chart of positive self-talk statements. Post it in the classroom and refer to it often. Make sure to notice when your classmates and you are using them. Is there a particular time of the day when you use them most often?

Learning Log

My goal this week: _____

_____

		Minutes Read:
Monday	_____ _____ _____ _____	_____
Tuesday	_____ _____ _____ _____	_____
Wednesday	_____ _____ _____ _____	_____
Thursday	_____ _____ _____ _____	_____
Friday	_____ _____ _____ _____	_____
Home/School Communication		

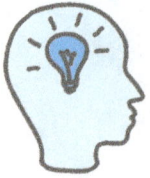

Identity and Mindset Review (Review # 1)

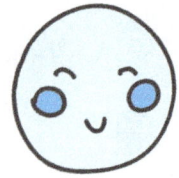

Reflection:

Look over the last nine lessons, from All About Me to Self-Talk. From those lessons, what is one thing that you've been thinking about and working on lately?

_____

_____

_____

What is something you'd like to start working on?

_____

_____

_____

As a class:

Take some time to do some of these activities:

Play the space bubble game. Pretend you are all in space bubbles, and try not to touch each other as you walk around the room! See if you can find ways of changing the game to make it more challenging.

Sing the version of "If You're Happy and You Know It" that you made up or make up a new version. As a class, decide on which emotion, words and movements/sounds you'll make for each emotion that has been covered after the first verse.

Play charades with emotions. After writing the emotions on cards, take turns acting them out and guessing. How can you show the difference between some similar emotions, like angry and frustrated?

Write skits to show ways to make friends and ask to play. Act them out for students in a class with younger students.

Learning Log

My goal this week: _____

_____

		Minutes Read:
Monday	_____ _____ _____ _____	_____
Tuesday	_____ _____ _____ _____	Minutes Read: _____
Wednesday	_____ _____ _____ _____	Minutes Read: _____
Thursday	_____ _____ _____ _____	Minutes Read: _____
Friday	_____ _____ _____ _____	Minutes Read: _____
Home/School Communication		

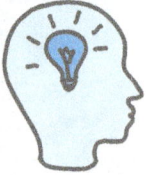

Goal Check-In

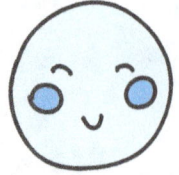

Look back at the goals you set for yourself at the beginning of the year. Write the number of two goals here and add notes to check in or make changes to your goals. It's ok to add to or change your goals a little, but keep pushing yourself to grow this year. If you feel you have met your goal, make a new goal for yourself at the bottom of this page.

Goal _____: *Circle one of the options below.*

I've completed this goal!   I'm still working on this goal.   I'm struggling with this goal and need help.

What I need to adjust or continue working on, and who can help me:_____

_____

Goal _____: *Circle one of the options below.*

I've completed this goal!   I'm still working on this goal.   I'm struggling with this goal and need help.

What I need to adjust or continue working on, and who can help me:_____

_____

New goal:

Goal _____: _____

_____

Date you will accomplish this goal: _____

Steps you will take to reach this goal: _____

_____

Who can you ask for help with this goal? _____

How will you know you've accomplished this goal? _____

_____

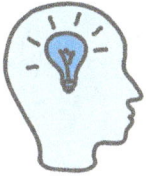

Social-Emotional Learning Connection

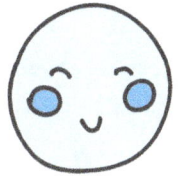

Think about a book you loved reading or listening to lately.

What was the title of the book? _____

What did you love about this book? Draw a picture or write your answer below.

How did the characters play and work together? What skills did you notice them using from our planner? (For example, maybe a character needed personal space and used their words to get the space they needed.) Draw or write your answers below.

Notes

Notes

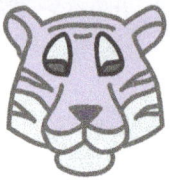

courage and kindness

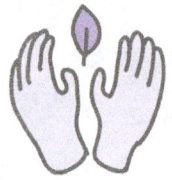

You have just finished the theme on identity and mindset, and we are now transitioning to courage and kindness with a focus on the social-emotional competency of relationship skills.

Throughout this theme, you will be learning about:

1. Listening to others (Teamwork & Social engagement)
2. Asking permission (Communication & Social engagement)
3. Saying no and accepting no (Communication & Relationship-building)
4. Speaking up (Social engagement)
5. Listening to your body and understanding mixed feelings (Self-Awareness competency & Social engagement)

Standing up for yourself and for others shows courage, but it also shows kindness and compassion to others. You and your carer can explore more about courage and kindness over the next ten weeks by reading books about these topics. Here's a list of some of the books you can check out at your school or community library to read together:

Peace is an Offering by Annette LeBox

Pass it On by Sophy Henn

Emma and the Whale by Julie Case

The Rabbit Listened by Cori Doerrfeld

Hey, Little Ant by Phillip Hoose

Adrian Simcox does NOT have a Horse by Marcy Campbell

Jabari Jumps by Gaia Cornwall

Come with Me by Holly M. McGhee

How to be a Lion by Ed Vere

One by Kathryn Otoshi

The Smallest Girl in the Smallest Grade by Justin Roberts

I Walk with Vanessa by Kerascoët

When You are Brave by Pat Zietlow Mille

Tomorrow I'll Be Brave by Jessica Hische

Shy by Deborah Freedman

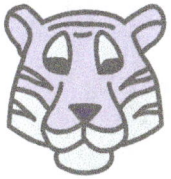

courage and kindness

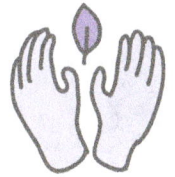

Color all the images that show a person displaying courage and bravery red.

Color all the images that show kindness with blue.

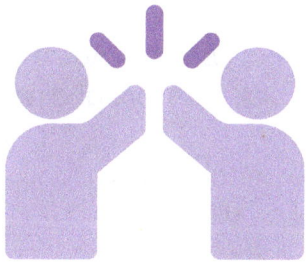

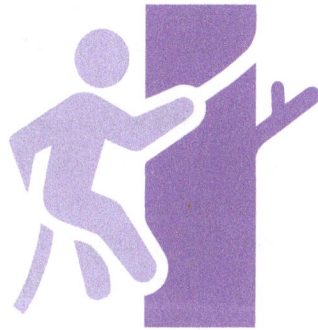

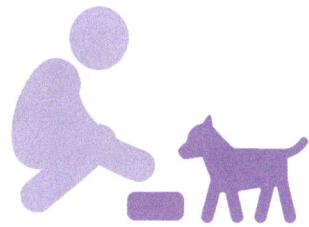

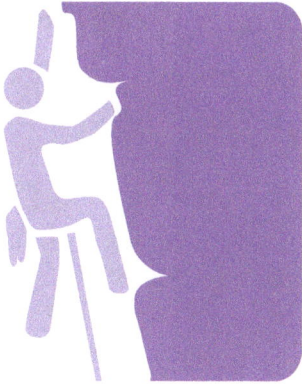

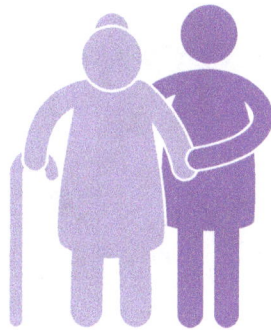

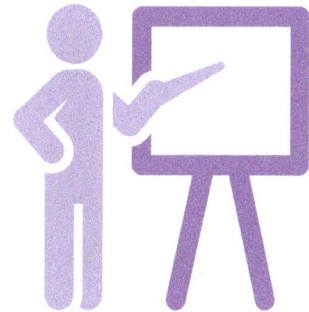

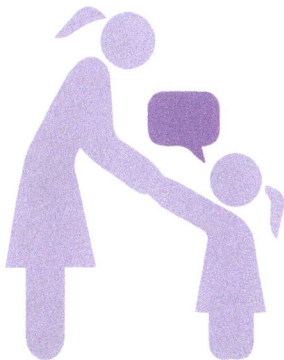

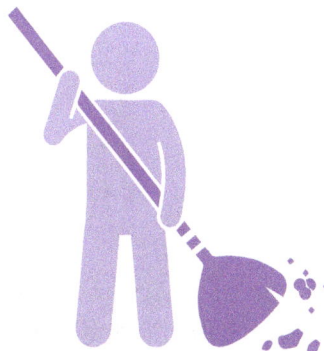

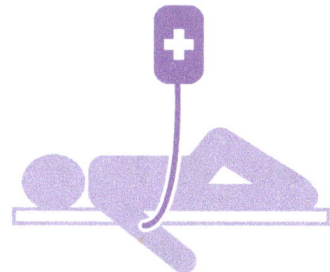

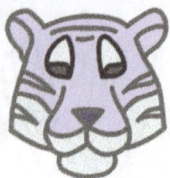

Active Listening

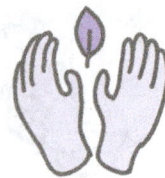

When talking to other people (friends, teachers, parents, etc.), it is important to be an active listener. That means you need to not only listen with your ears, but show you are listening in other ways, too. Sometimes, people even call active listening 'whole body listening' because you can use your whole body to show you're listening. In whole body listening, you use the following body parts in these ways:

- Eyes—Look at the person who is talking to you. Make eye contact and notice other ways in which the person is communicating, with facial expressions and gestures, etc.
- Ears—Listen to what is being said.
- Brain—Think about the big ideas of what the person is saying, not just the words.
- Mouth—It is good to stay quiet while the other person speaks. Ask questions and repeat back what is being said when you can.
- Shoulders—Keep your shoulders and body turned toward the person who is talking.
- Heart—Respect and care about what the person is saying.
- Hands and feet—Keep your hands and feet still.

Practice:
Label the parts of the body that are used for active listening and what you do with them. See the example below.

Hands and feet –
Keep still

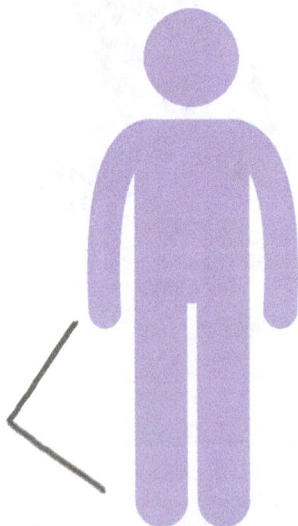

Extension:
In small groups, play the Telephone game. Whisper a message to one person, who will whisper it to another person, who will whisper it to the next person. When the final person gets the message, they will say it aloud to see how similar or different it is from the original message. Why do you think the message is different from the original message? Which aspects of active listening did you use in this game? Would the use of other aspects of active listening help improve the message? Try to design a game that could test that.

Learning Log

My goal this week: _____

_____

		Minutes Read:
Monday	_____ _____ _____ _____	_____
Tuesday	_____ _____ _____ _____	Minutes Read: _____
Wednesday	_____ _____ _____ _____	Minutes Read: _____
Thursday	_____ _____ _____ _____	Minutes Read: _____
Friday	_____ _____ _____ _____	Minutes Read: _____
Home/School Communication		

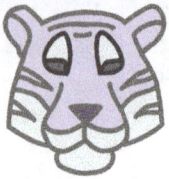

Asking Permission

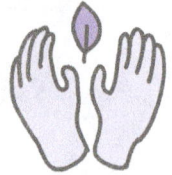

When we want to do something, we need to ask permission to do it. Asking permission means we are asking the person who is in charge if they will allow us to do, use, or have something. Some examples of when we ask permission are to go to the bathroom during school, to use someone else's pencil or toy, or to hug another person. We ask permission to show respect for rules, people's belongings, or people's boundaries or bodies. Words used to ask permission to do something are, "May I...." or "Can I...". An example is, "May I please use your red marker?".

Practice:

Write the words you would use to ask permission in these situations.

You forgot your homework in your backpack, which is in your cubby.

_____

_____

You see your best friend for the first time after summer vacation. You are so excited to see her that you want to give her a hug. How do you ask permission?

_____

_____

You are about to complete a painting. You only have a thick paintbrush, but see that your classmate has a thin one that would be perfect. How will you ask permission to use it?

_____

_____

Extension:

Play a different form of the game "Mother, May I?", called "Friend, May I?". Choose someone to be the Friend. Have the Friend stand on one side of the room with their back toward the rest of the children. At the other end of the room, the other children line up next to each other. Children take turns asking, "Friend, may I take (number) (type of) steps?" The Friend can say "Yes, you may" or "No, you may not". If they say no, another option may be given; for example, "No, but you may take (number) (type of) steps." Possible types of steps are giant steps, baby steps, regular steps, scissor steps, bunny hops, frog hops. The first child to reach the Friend becomes the next Friend. After playing, talk about why the Friend might give permission for only some types of steps.

Learning Log

My goal this week: _____

_____

		Minutes Read:
Monday	_____ _____ _____ _____	_____
Tuesday	_____ _____ _____ _____	Minutes Read: _____
Wednesday	_____ _____ _____ _____	Minutes Read: _____
Thursday	_____ _____ _____ _____	Minutes Read: _____
Friday	_____ _____ _____ _____	Minutes Read: _____
Home/School Communication		

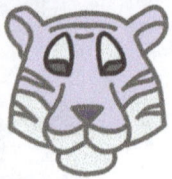

Listening to Your Body

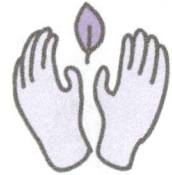

It is important for us to think about our own bodies and how they can tell us the way we are feeling. This can be done by listening to our bodies' signals. This is not just about listening with our ears like we listen to music. It is thinking about how different parts of our body are giving us signals that tell us our emotions. Here are some signals in different parts of the body that you should pay attention to:

- Breath: Is it fast or slow? Is it deep or shallow?
- Heartbeat: Is it fast or slow? Is it pounding or calm?
- Belly: Is it soft, turning, or tight?
- Muscles: Are they tense or relaxed?
- Energy Level: Are you tired or energetic? Calm or wiggly?
- Temperature: Are you hot or cold?
- Other signals: Are you hungry? Thirsty? Full? Comfortable?

Once you notice these signals, think about what they are trying to tell you. What emotion are you feeling? What do you need right now?

Practice:
Take a minute to close your eyes and think about how all these body parts and functions feel right now. Then, fill in the chart. Next, do 20 jumping jacks. Then sit down, close your eyes and again think about each of these body parts/functions feels. Again, fill in the chart. This will give you an idea about how the different signals can feel.

	Right now	After jumping jacks
Breath		
Heartbeat		
Belly		
Muscles		
Energy Level		
Temperature		
Other signals		

Extension:
Talk to a partner about which signals might connect with which emotion. For example, how would your breath and heartbeat feel if you are angry? Make a list of which signals might connect with which emotions.

Learning Log

My goal this week: _____

_____

		Minutes Read:
Monday	_____ _____ _____ _____	_____
Tuesday	_____ _____ _____ _____	Minutes Read: _____
Wednesday	_____ _____ _____ _____	Minutes Read: _____
Thursday	_____ _____ _____ _____	Minutes Read: _____
Friday	_____ _____ _____ _____	Minutes Read: _____
Home/School Communication		

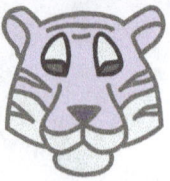

Regulating Your Emotions

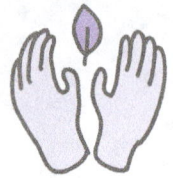

We know about different emotions, some strategies to use when we feel those emotions, and how to listen to our bodies to understand which emotion we're feeling. This is important because our emotions affect our behavior and our behavior can affect our learning. While it is always OK to feel how we feel, we want to make sure that those feelings do not affect our relationships and learning. One way to help with this is to try to regulate, or control, the amount we feel an emotion, so that it doesn't overpower everything else we would like to do. One of the best tools we can use to regulate our emotions is to belly breathe. This can help the emotion we're feeling to not feel as big. While it will still be there, we can take our time and think about what we want to do about it instead of reacting thoughtlessly.

Steps for belly breathing:
Put your hands on your belly.
Breathe in slowly, filling up your belly, while counting to 4.
Hold your breath for 4 counts.
Breathe out slowly, counting to 4.
Repeat.

Try this when you're feeling big emotions. Then you can think about what you need to do next.

Practice:
Try a different way of breathing, called bunny breathing. Sit on your knees. Take three quick breaths in through your nose, like a bunny sniffing. Breathe out slowly through your mouth. Repeat.

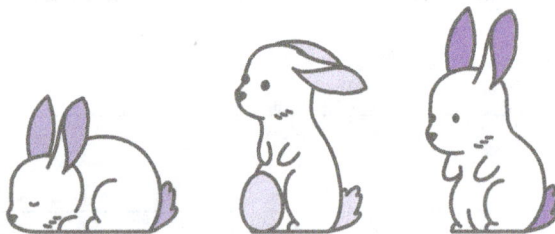

Which type of breathing do you prefer—the belly breathing or the bunny breathing? Why?

_____

_____

Extension:
Create a new way of breathing and share it with your class. For example, what would dragon breathing look like? Taco breathing?

Learning Log

My goal this week: _____

_____

		Minutes Read:
Monday	_____ _____ _____ _____	_____
Tuesday	_____ _____ _____ _____	Minutes Read: _____
Wednesday	_____ _____ _____ _____	Minutes Read: _____
Thursday	_____ _____ _____ _____	Minutes Read: _____
Friday	_____ _____ _____ _____	Minutes Read: _____
Home/School Communication		

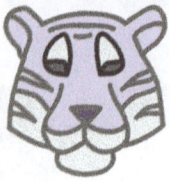

Mixed feelings

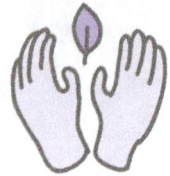

Sometimes, we feel more than just one emotion at a time. For example, when we do something new, we can feel both nervous and excited. When we have such feelings, we can say that we have mixed feelings. It is OK to have mixed feelings. As with any emotion, we need to think about what we're feeling by listening to what our body is telling us and then think about what we should do next.

Practice:

When was a time that you had mixed feelings?

_____

_____

_____

What feelings did you have?

_____

What did you do?

_____

_____

_____

Can you predict when you might have mixed feelings?

_____

_____

_____

Extension:
Make some art to reflect what it feels like to have mixed feelings. It can be a painting, a drawing, a sculpture or any other form of art. Give it a title and write a description of what it means to you.

Learning Log

My goal this week: _____

_____

		Minutes Read:
Monday	_____ _____ _____ _____	Minutes Read: _____
Tuesday	_____ _____ _____ _____	Minutes Read: _____
Wednesday	_____ _____ _____ _____	Minutes Read: _____
Thursday	_____ _____ _____ _____	Minutes Read: _____
Friday	_____ _____ _____ _____	Minutes Read: _____
Home/School Communication		

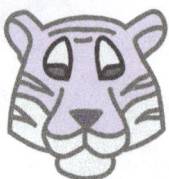

COLORING PAGE

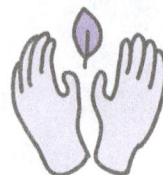

Use your finger or a crayon to trace the 8 below. As you trace, practice your breathing by breathing in while you trace the top part of the 8, then breathe out while you trace the bottom part of the 8. Can you breathe slowly like this eight times while you trace and color?

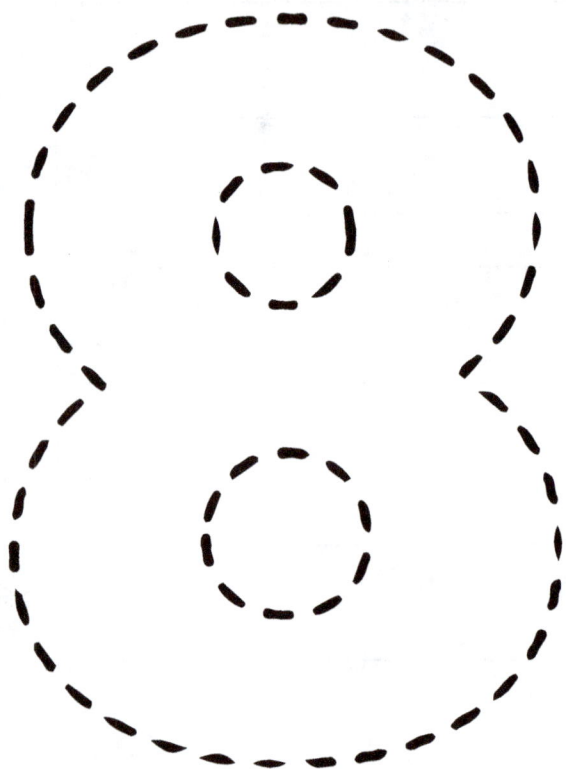

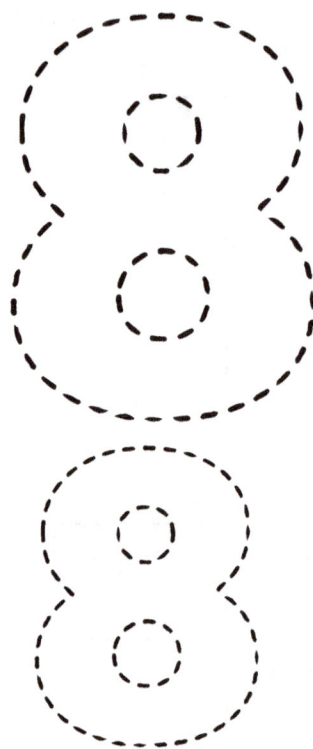

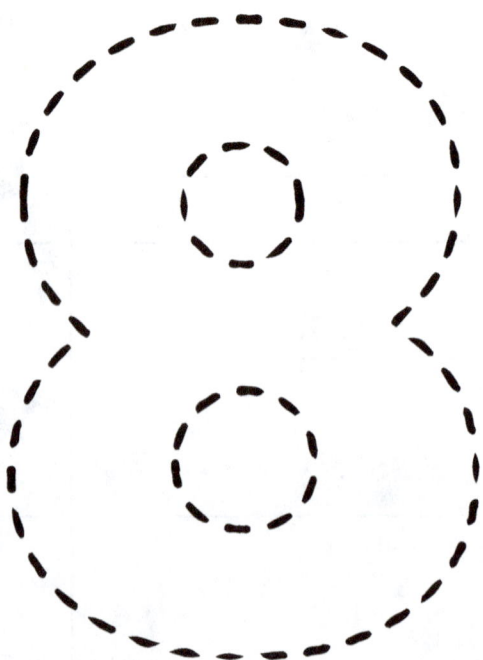

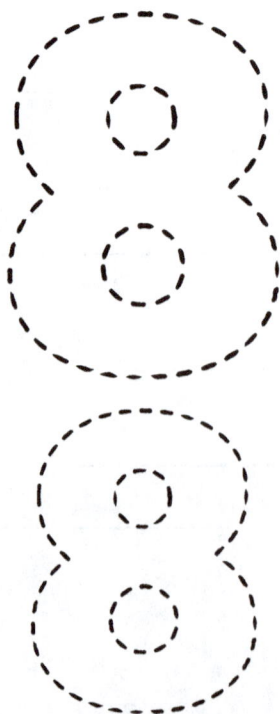

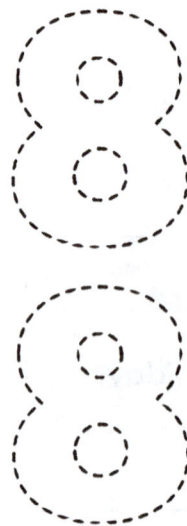

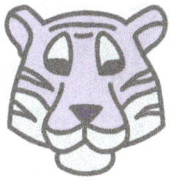

COLORING PAGE

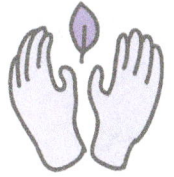

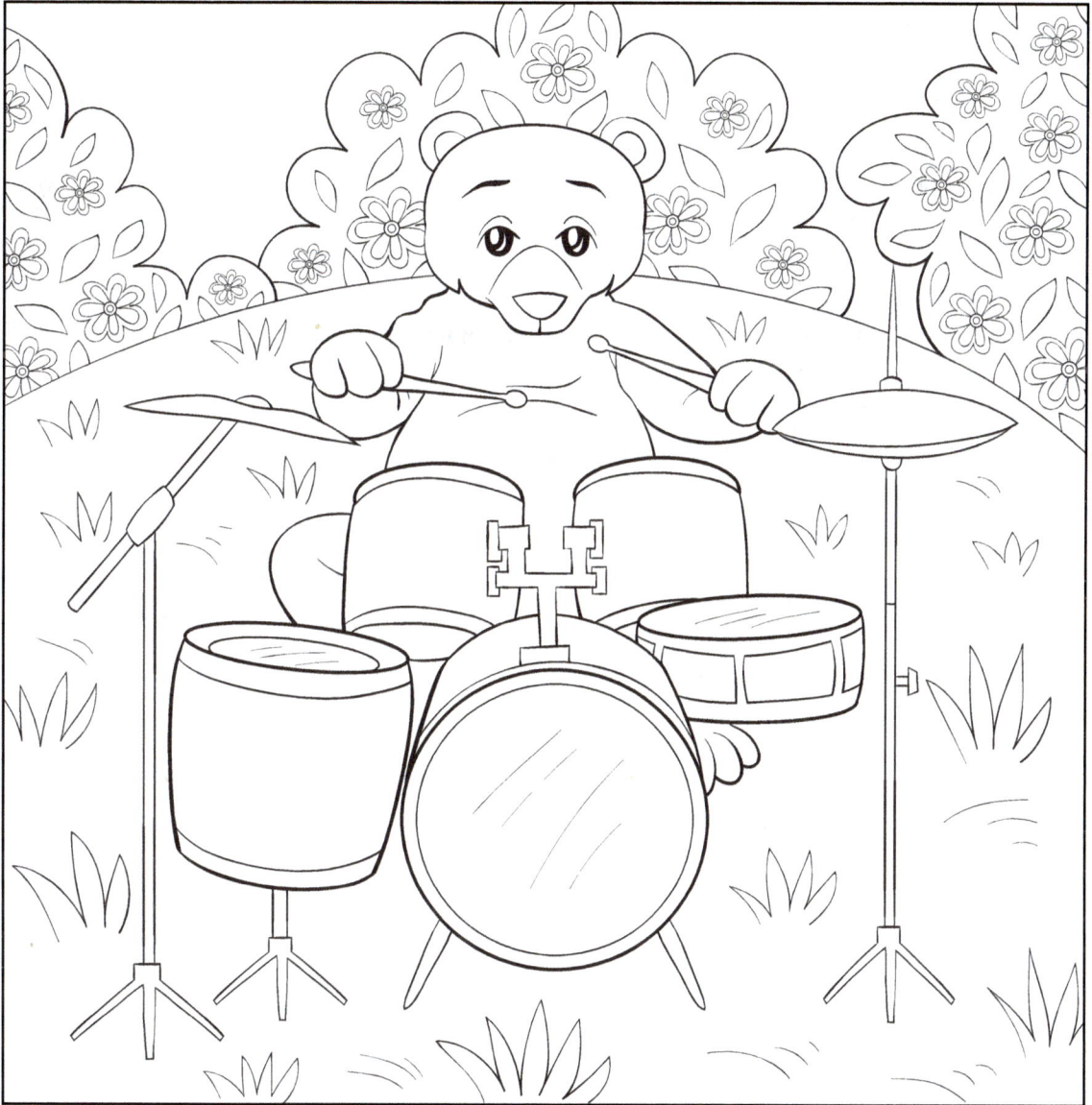

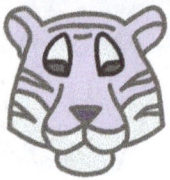

Saying No

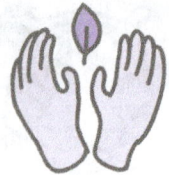

At home and in school, you have probably learned that it is important to follow instructions and that it is not usually OK for you to say no when your parent or carer or teacher asks you to do something. But there are some times when it is very important to say no. Some examples of times when you should say no are when someone takes something from you, someone is in your personal space or touching you, or someone asks you to do something that makes you feel uncomfortable or unsafe. When you find yourself in such a situation, you should look at the person you're talking to and say no in a firm voice. You might give a reason why you don't like what is happening or don't want to do what is being asked. Or, you might just go away to a different place. If you ever have to tell someone no because they did something that made you feel uncomfortable, you should always tell an adult you trust what happened.

Practice:
For the situations written below, write **no** in the blank if you think it is important to say no in that situation.

_____ Your mom asks you to clean your room.

_____ Your classmate squeezes in to sit next to you on the same chair.

_____ Your brother tells you to climb onto the counter to reach something high up.

_____ Your teacher tells you to write your name on your homework.

_____ Your friend grabs the Lego tower you built to add more Legos to it.

_____ Your classmate tells you to cut another classmate's hair with scissors.

_____ Your teacher asks you to line up to go to lunch.

_____ At the park, an adult that you don't know asks to take a picture of you.

Extension:
In small groups, role play situations in which you need to say no. You can use some of the situations written above or make your own situations. Talk about these questions in your group: How do you feel once you say no? Is it easier to say no to some people than others? Who is it hardest to say no to? Why do you think that is?

Learning Log

My goal this week: _____

_____

		Minutes Read:
Monday	_____ _____ _____ _____	_____
Tuesday	_____ _____ _____ _____	_____
Wednesday	_____ _____ _____ _____	_____
Thursday	_____ _____ _____ _____	_____
Friday	_____ _____ _____ _____	_____
Home/School Communication		

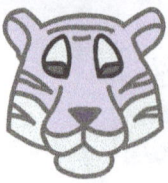

Speaking Up

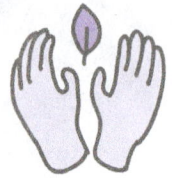

As we learned, there are times when it is important to say no for ourselves. It is also important for us to speak up when we see unfair or unsafe things happening to others. For example, if we see that someone is treating another person in an unkind way or doing something unsafe, we need to speak up by looking at the person, using a firm voice, and telling whoever is behaving unkindly to stop. If that doesn't work, then we need to get an adult to help. If we don't speak up when we see something unfair or unkind happening, then we could be part of the problem.

Practice:
Write the words you would use to speak up in the situations written below.

You notice that one of your classmates is taking food off of another classmate's tray every day at lunch.

_____

_____

_____

There is a new student in your class who has just moved here from another country. You hear some other students making fun of the way they dress.

_____

_____

_____

A student in your class has a little trouble saying some words. You hear other students making fun of and imitating the way they speak.

_____

_____

_____

Extension:
Use puppets to act out some situations in which you need to speak up for others. Think about whether you also need to get help from adults in those situations. Is it easier to speak up in some situations than others? What makes it difficult to speak up sometimes? Is there something you can do to make it easier?

Learning Log

My goal this week: _____

_____

		Minutes Read:
Monday	_____ _____ _____ _____	_____
Tuesday	_____ _____ _____ _____	Minutes Read: _____
Wednesday	_____ _____ _____ _____	Minutes Read: _____
Thursday	_____ _____ _____ _____	Minutes Read: _____
Friday	_____ _____ _____ _____	Minutes Read: _____
Home/School Communication		

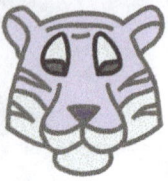

Seeking Help

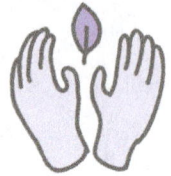

When you are working on something and feel like you are stuck, what should you do? You can ask for help. In general, this is how you politely ask for help: "Could you help me, please?"

It is important to ask for help when you need it, but you should first think carefully about what help you need. Here are some things to think about when you are going to ask for help:

- What resources are available to get help?
- Can you ask a classmate to help you with what you need?
- Do you actually need help or do you just need some more time to think?
- Is now a good time to ask for help from your teacher?
- Be specific about what help you need. "I can't do this." or "I don't understand." are not useful ways of asking for help.
    - What have you already tried? Explain this when asking for help. "I tried _____ and _____, but I am still having trouble. Could you please help me?"
    - What parts do you understand? What parts are you confused about? Explain that when asking for help.

Practice:

Match the situations shown on the left with the ideas to ask for help on the right.

1. _____ Leilani is working on her math homework. She has solved the first four problems, but she is having trouble with the fifth one.	A. "I have tried putting the wheels on like this and putting the blocks together like this, but it keeps falling apart. Could you please help me?"
2. _____ Sudipta has all of the pieces of the craft he's going to assemble in front of him, but he doesn't know what to do first.	B. Ask a classmate to remind you of the instructions.
3. _____ Noor is working on building a car out of magnetic blocks, but it keeps collapsing.	C. Read the instructions that you have in front of you.
4. _____ Dwayne is working on a science activity with his group and he is not sure what he is supposed to do next.	D. "I read the problem and I know that I need to add the numbers, but I am not sure which ones I need to add. Could you please help me?"

Extension:

As a class, make a chart with ideas for how to get help when needed. Make sure that you use students' own words. Students could take photos of each other acting out ways to get help to add to the chart or make illustrations. When necessary, refer to the chart.

Learning Log

My goal this week: _____

_____

Monday	_____ _____	Minutes Read: _____
Tuesday	_____ _____	Minutes Read: _____
Wednesday	_____ _____	Minutes Read: _____
Thursday	_____ _____	Minutes Read: _____
Friday	_____ _____	Minutes Read: _____
Home/School Communication		

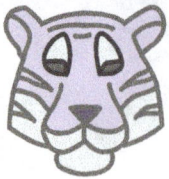

Accepting No

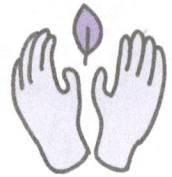

We learned how important it is to sometimes say no to other people. It is also important for us to accept when someone says no to us. It can be hard when we ask someone for something or to do something, and their answer is 'no.' But we need to learn how to accept such an answer. When we get a no, we need to look at the person and say OK. It is important to stay calm in the moment. If we disagree with the answer, it is something that we can bring up and discuss at another time, not argue about right then.

Usually, there is a reason why a person has answered no to what we have asked. Most people don't want to keep talking about it and arguing about it. No means no and we need to move on.

Practice:
Think about a time when someone told you no. Think about a time when someone told you no. What did you say to accept it?

_____

_____

_____

Was there ever a time when someone told you no and you got upset? What happened next?

_____

_____

_____

Extension:
In small groups, role play some situations in which you need to accept a no answer. Here are some suggestions:

• Ask your teacher to go to the bathroom. She tells you no; you can go in 10 minutes when it is lunch time.
• Ask your dad if you can watch one more show on TV. He says no.
• Ask your parents if you can walk to your friend's house by yourself. They say no.
• Ask your friend if you can have one of his cookies. He says no.

Are there times when it is easier to accept a no answer? What makes it easier?

Learning Log

My goal this week: _____

_____

		Minutes Read:
Monday	_____ _____ _____ _____	_____
Tuesday	_____ _____ _____ _____	Minutes Read: _____
Wednesday	_____ _____ _____ _____	Minutes Read: _____
Thursday	_____ _____ _____ _____	Minutes Read: _____
Friday	_____ _____ _____ _____	Minutes Read: _____
Home/School Communication		

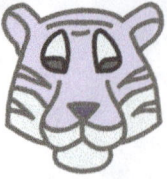

Courage and Kindness Review
(Review # 2)

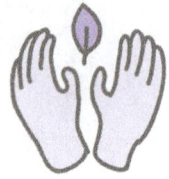

Reflection:

Look over the last nine lessons, from Active Listening to Accepting No. What is one thing that you've been thinking about and working on lately?

_____

_____

_____

What is something you'd like to start working on?

_____

_____

_____

As a class:

Take some time out to do some of the activities mentioned below:

Play the Telephone game. Whisper a message to one person, who will whisper it to another person, who, in turn, will whisper it to the next person. When the final person gets the message, they will say it aloud to find out how similar or different it is from the original message.

Play "Friend, May I?" See the lesson on 'Asking Permission' for directions.

Take some time to listen to your body. Think about the signals you're feeling. What emotions are you feeling? Talk with a partner about what you're feeling and the emotion that it connects to.

Practice one of the breathing techniques—belly breathing or bunny breathing—or another breathing technique you know.

Write skits to show ways of saying no and for speaking up for others. Act them out for students in a class with younger students.

Learning Log

My goal this week: _____

_____

		Minutes Read:
Monday	_____ _____ _____ _____	Minutes Read: _____
Tuesday	_____ _____ _____ _____	Minutes Read: _____
Wednesday	_____ _____ _____ _____	Minutes Read: _____
Thursday	_____ _____ _____ _____	Minutes Read: _____
Friday	_____ _____ _____ _____	Minutes Read: _____
Home/School Communication		

Goal Check-In

Look back at the goals you set for yourself at the beginning of the year or the last Goal Check-In. Write the number of two goals here and add notes to check in or make changes to your goals. It's ok to add to or change your goals a little, but keep pushing yourself to grow this year. If you feel you have met your goal, make a new goal for yourself at the bottom of this page.

Goal _____: *Circle one of the options below.*

I've completed this goal!   I'm still working on this goal.   I'm struggling with this goal and need help.

What I need to adjust or continue working on, and who can help me:_____

_____

Goal _____: *Circle one of the options below.*

I've completed this goal!   I'm still working on this goal.   I'm struggling with this goal and need help.

What I need to adjust or continue working on, and who can help me:_____

_____

New goal:

Goal _____: _____

_____

Date you will accomplish this goal: _____

Steps you will take to reach this goal: _____

_____

Who can you ask for help with this goal? _____

How will you know you've accomplished this goal? _____

_____

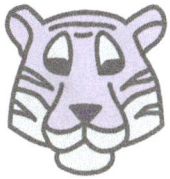

Social-Emotional Learning Connection

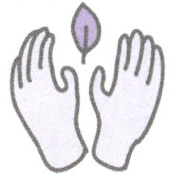

Think about a book you loved reading or listening to lately.

What was the title of the book? _____

What did you love about this book? Draw a picture or write your answer below.

What types of emotions did the characters feel throughout the book?

How did the characters regulate (or not regulate) their emotions? Did any of the characters use some of the tools we've discussed in our SEL Planner over the last 20 weeks? What tools did they use? Draw or write your answers below.

Notes

Notes

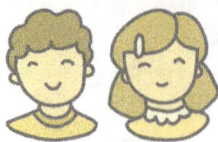

A Place to Belong

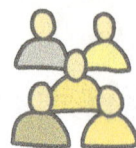

Belonging is a vital element of being human. We all want a place to belong and as humans we also have the opportunity to help others feel a sense of belonging. These next 10 weeks we will focus on the idea of belonging with an emphasis on the social-emotional competency of social-awareness.

Throughout this theme, you will be exploring:
1. Other cultures (Appreciating diversity & Respect for others)
2. Cooperation and disagreeing respectfully(Empathy & Perspective-taking)
3. Lifting others up (Appreciating diversity, Respect for others, & Perspective-taking)
4. Apologizing and maintaining friendships (Self-Awareness competency)
5. Giving and accepting compliments (Empathy, Respect for others, & Self-Awareness competency)

You can read stories about belonging by checking out the books below from your local or school library, and reading them to yourself or with your carer. The book list below includes books about a range of different people and locations. Reading is a way to travel and learn about new people and places without leaving your hometown! Enjoy these books!

Most People by Michael Leannah
The Masterpiece (One Big Canvas) by Jay Miletsky
Lovely by Jess Hong
Why Am I Me? By Paige Britt
Last Stop on Market Street by Matt de la Peña
The Invisible Boy by Trudy Ludwig
All Are Welcome by Alexandra Penfold
Those Shoes by Maribeth Boelts
Explorers of the Wild by Cale Atkinson
The Name Jar by Yangsook Choi
Drawn Together by Minh Lê
Noah Chases the Wind by Michelle Worthington
The Big Umbrella by Amy June Bates
Here We are by Oliver Jeffers

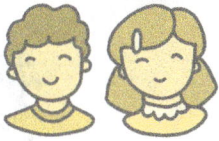

A Place to Belong

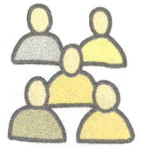

How does it feel when you belong somewhere?

_____

_____

_____

_____

Draw a picture of you somewhere you belong, including people you belong with.

I belong _____

with _____

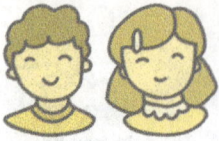

Celebrating Differences

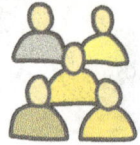

Think back to our very first lesson. We talked about how every person is unique and special. You thought of all the things that make you unique. If you think about it, you will find that while some of those things are similar to those of other people, other things are different. It is so special that we live in a world where each person is different and unique. Being around people who are different from us allows us to experience and learn new things. Sometimes, you may not understand the way that other people do things, since it is different from how you do things. You can ask, in a respectful way, for example, "In my family, we _____. I was wondering how you _____?" or "At home, I have to _____. What chores do you have to do?" The most important thing to understand is that everyone is different in some ways and does things differently. This means that no one way is the right way or the only way to do things.

Practice:

Work with a classmate to see if you can find some things that make you different from each other. First, fill in the left side of the chart with information only about you. Then, ask a classmate the questions, so you can fill in the right side of the chart with their information. Next, talk about the things that are different and the same.

Question	Your Name:	Classmate's Name:
What is the color of your eyes?		
Where do you live?		
Who lives with you?		
What is your favorite book to read?		
What do you like to do in your free time?		
What is your favorite food?		
What is something that your family likes to do together?		

Extension:

Work as a class to make some sort of display (writing, artwork, etc.) in order to celebrate things that make each student unique and special. Put it up somewhere in the classroom or the hallway to show off how these differences in each student make the class special. While you're working, reflect on what new things you learned about your classmates.

Learning Log

My goal this week: _____

_____

		Minutes Read:
Monday	_____ _____ _____ _____	_____
Tuesday	_____ _____ _____ _____	Minutes Read: _____
Wednesday	_____ _____ _____ _____	Minutes Read: _____
Thursday	_____ _____ _____ _____	Minutes Read: _____
Friday	_____ _____ _____ _____	Minutes Read: _____
Home/School Communication		

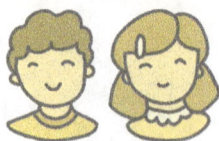

Disagreeing Respectfully

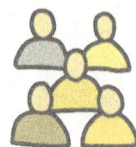

There are times when we agree with others, but there are also times when we disagree with them. When we don't agree, it is important for us to disagree in a respectful way so we do not hurt anyone's feelings. In order to do this, we can use "I" statements to explain what we are thinking and feeling instead of assuming that we already know what the other person is thinking and feeling. Some examples are:

"I disagree because…"

"I see what you're saying, but I wonder…"

"I hear what you think. Can you tell me why you think that?"

"I've listened to your idea; now can I share mine?"

In these examples, we let the other person know that we have listened to them. Then, we provide evidence to support our own opinion, ask questions, or offer an opinion.

Practice:
Write what you would say to disagree in a respectful way.

You and your classmate have both solved a math problem. Your answer is 52 miles. She says, "The answer is 32 miles." What would you say?

_____

_____

_____

Your little brother keeps telling you that there is a monster in his closet. What would you say?

_____

_____

_____

Your teacher asks you to make a drawing of the park. She says that the grass must be green and the sky must be blue. You would like to be creative and use different colors. What do you say?

_____

_____

_____

Extension: Work as a class to make a chart of sentence starters that can be used in discussions for agreeing and disagreeing with classmates in a respectful way. Post it in a location where it can be seen and made use of during class discussions.

Learning Log

My goal this week: _____

_____

		Minutes Read:
Monday	_____ _____ _____ _____	_____
Tuesday	_____ _____ _____ _____	Minutes Read: _____
Wednesday	_____ _____ _____ _____	Minutes Read: _____
Thursday	_____ _____ _____ _____	Minutes Read: _____
Friday	_____ _____ _____ _____	Minutes Read: _____
Home/School Communication		

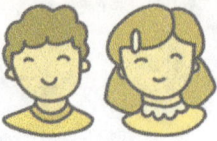

Conflict Resolution

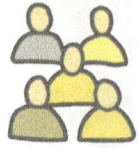

Sometimes, when playing or working together, we have conflicts. Conflicts are disagreements or problems we have with other people. It is important to use our words to resolve conflicts in a calm, peaceful way. To do that, we need to be calm, and every person must be allowed to speak while the other person listens. Here are some steps that can be used to resolve conflicts:

Person 1 explains the problem, using an "I" statement.
I didn't like it when you drew on my paper because now you can't see what I wrote.

Person 2 says what they heard Person 1 say.
I heard that you didn't like it when I drew on your paper because now you can't see the writing.

Person 2 has a chance to explain their actions.
I didn't mean to draw on your paper. I was trying to reach the marker top and I wasn't paying attention to where the marker was.

Together, both people figure out a solution for the problem.
What if I tell the teacher that I drew on your paper by accident and ask her if she can still figure out what it says?

After agreeing on a solution, whatever was decided needs to be done.

Practice:
What words would Sofia and Jacob use to resolve their conflict?
<u>Conflict:</u> Jacob asks Sofia if he can join in the game of freeze tag she is playing with a group of friends on the playground. Instead of answering, Sofia just runs away.

Jacob   **Sofia**

Jacob   **Sofia**

Jacob   **Sofia**

Extension: Use puppets to act out conflicts and resolve them.

Learning Log

My goal this week: _____

_____

Monday	_____ _____ _____ _____	Minutes Read: _____
Tuesday	_____ _____ _____ _____	Minutes Read: _____
Wednesday	_____ _____ _____ _____	Minutes Read: _____
Thursday	_____ _____ _____ _____	Minutes Read: _____
Friday	_____ _____ _____ _____	Minutes Read: _____
Home/School Communication		

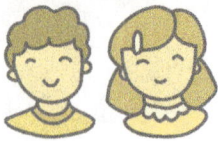

Apologizing

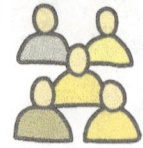

It is important to apologize, or to say sorry, when we have done something wrong. Since simply saying "I'm sorry" doesn't make it right, it is important that apology is thoughtful and considers how you can repair the harm that has been done. Make sure that you look the person in the eye when apologizing.

Steps to an Apology::
   "I'm sorry for…" (say what you did that was wrong)
   "It was wrong because…" (why were your actions hurtful)
   "What can I do to make it better?"
   "Next time I will…" (what you WILL do differently next time, do NOT say what you won't do next time)
   You may wish to ask for forgiveness by saying, "Will you forgive me?"

When someone apologizes to you, you need to look the person in the eye and listen to what they are saying. You can help them come up with ideas that can make it better. Finally, you can accept the apology in many ways. Some ideas of what you could say are:
   "I accept your apology"
   "I forgive you"
   "Thank you for telling me"
   "We are still friends"

Practice:
Imagine that you need to apologize to your friend for taking her pencil. What should you say?

_____

_____

_____

_____

_____

Extension:
Practice apologizing and accepting apologies with a partner. Why is it important to use all of the steps instead of just saying I'm sorry? Which step of apologizing is the most difficult for you? How can you make it easier?

Learning Log

My goal this week: _____

_____

		Minutes Read:
Monday	_____ _____ _____ _____	_____
Tuesday	_____ _____ _____ _____	_____
Wednesday	_____ _____ _____ _____	_____
Thursday	_____ _____ _____ _____	_____
Friday	_____ _____ _____ _____	_____
Home/School Communication		

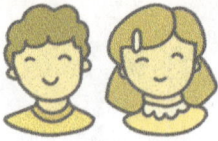

Compromising

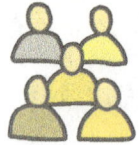

Sometimes, we need to compromise when we are working or playing with a group of people. To compromise means to come to an agreement that doesn't give everyone exactly what they want, but works for the group as a whole. For example, you and your friend are trying to decide what game to play. If you want to play superheroes but your friend wants to play soccer, then you need to compromise. You can each ask the other person if they would like to play what you want to play. If they say no, try to find something that you both would like to play. In this case, the two of you will maybe decide that you'd both be happy to play freeze tag together. Another way to compromise would be to decide to play one game first and the other later.

Practice:

How could the people in the following scenarios compromise?

Chan wants to stay at the park, but his sister wants to go home now.

_____

_____

_____

Sandra wants to play Candyland, but Analia wants to play Guess Who?.

_____

_____

_____

Natalie and Jason are working on a project at school. Natalie wants to make a poster, but Jason wants to make a book.

_____

_____

_____

Extension:

Work with a small group to role play compromise. Then, discuss questions such as: What did you do to help compromise? What did it feel like to compromise? What might you do differently next time?

Learning Log

My goal this week: _____

_____

		Minutes Read:
Monday	_____ _____ _____ _____	Minutes Read: _____
Tuesday	_____ _____ _____ _____	Minutes Read: _____
Wednesday	_____ _____ _____ _____	Minutes Read: _____
Thursday	_____ _____ _____ _____	Minutes Read: _____
Friday	_____ _____ _____ _____	Minutes Read: _____
Home/School Communication		

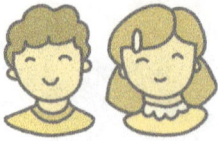 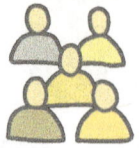

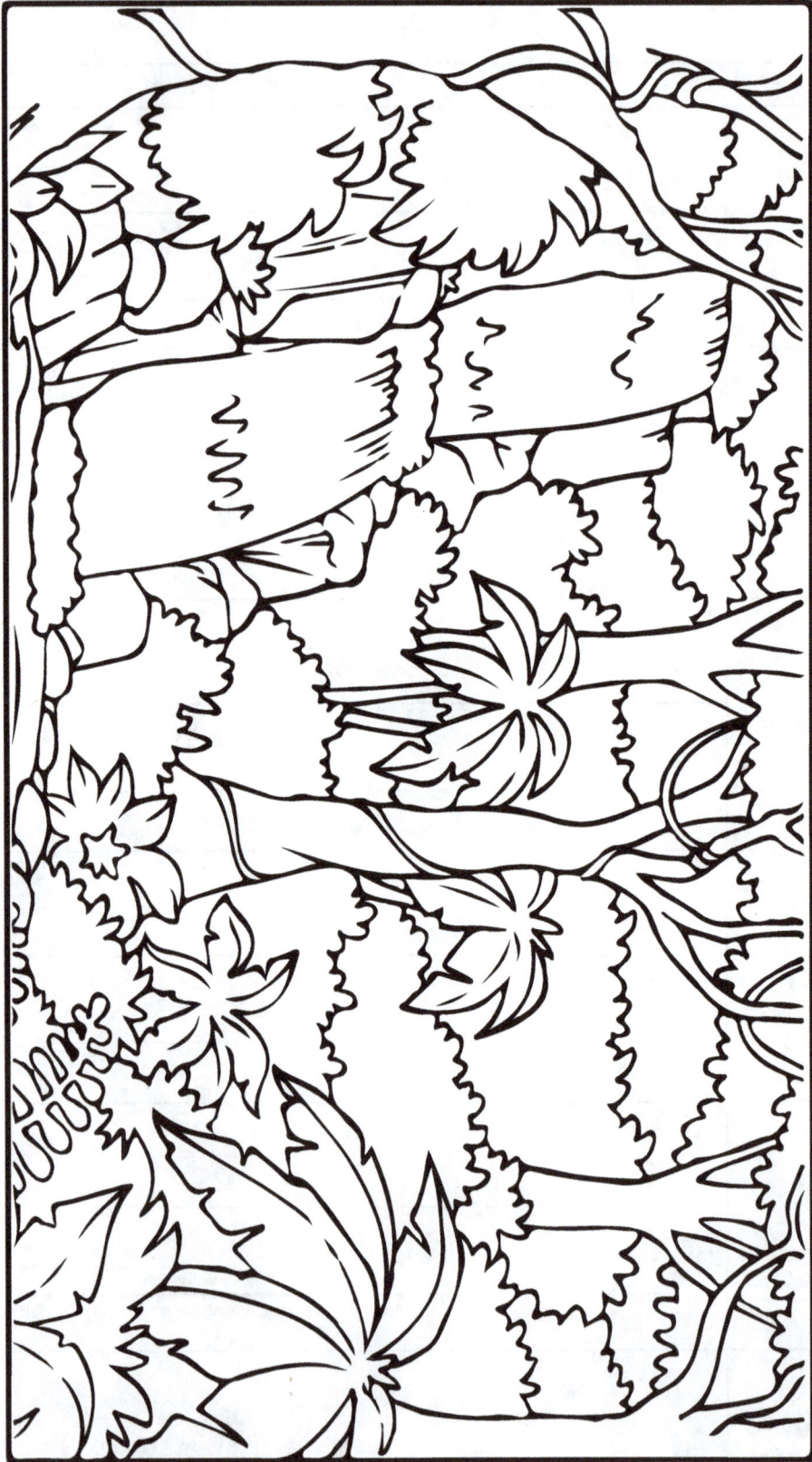

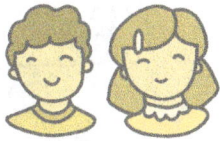

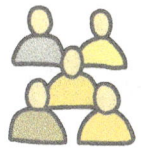

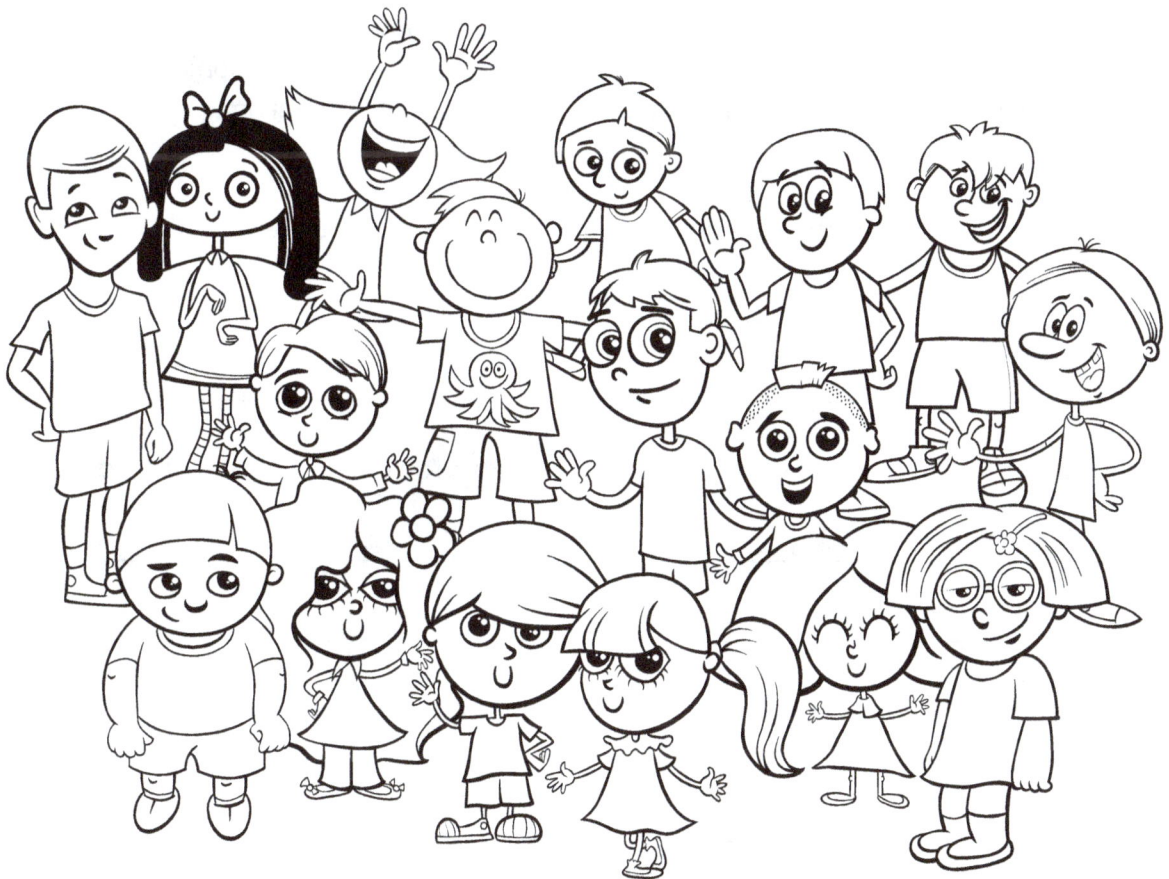

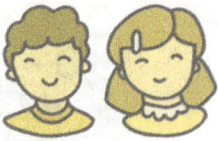

Maintaining Friendships

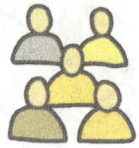

In one of our first lessons, we talked about making friends. You've had a lot of time in school now to make friends and practice many of the skills that you've learned so far. In addition to the skills you've already learned, you can do some other things to help maintain or keep friendships.

When playing, one of the best rules you can use is "You can't say you can't play," which comes from Vivian Paley, a preschool and kindergarten teacher. With this rule, there is never any reason to say no when someone asks if they can play with you. You can always find a way to compromise and play together. If you follow this rule, everyone feels included and part of the group.

Another thing you can do when playing and working with friends is to take turns. If you do that, everyone can have a turn instead of only one person having a turn. Sometimes, you will have to wait for your turn, which means that you will have to be patient.

Practice:
Has anyone ever told you that you can't play? How did it make you feel?

_____

_____

Why do you think it is important to have a rule that says, "You can't say you can't play"?

_____

_____

How can the rule "You can't say you can't play" and taking turns help you to maintain friendships?

_____

_____

Extension:
Make some posters of the rule "You can't say you can't play." Hang them in your classroom to remind you and your classmates of the rule or take them to other classrooms and teach other students about why the rule is important.

Learning Log

My goal this week: _____

_____

		Minutes Read:
Monday	_____ _____ _____ _____	_____
Tuesday	_____ _____ _____ _____	Minutes Read: _____
Wednesday	_____ _____ _____ _____	Minutes Read: _____
Thursday	_____ _____ _____ _____	Minutes Read: _____
Friday	_____ _____ _____ _____	Minutes Read: _____
Home/School Communication		

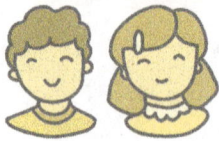

cooperation

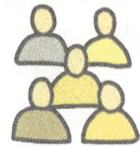

Cooperation happens when people work together to do something. There are many times in school, at home, when you are on a team, and when you are working in a group that you need to cooperate with other people. In order to cooperate with others, you need to talk to each other about what you're doing. You need to make a plan and work together. You should also make sure that each person has the opportunity to do something, so it is important to take turns and share.

Practice:
Cooperate with a partner to draw a picture of what it looks like to work with others. Have each partner use a different writing tool.

What worked well when you were cooperating to do your drawing? What didn't work? What could you do differently next time you're trying to cooperate?

_____

_____

_____

Extension:
Play a game with a parachute and lots of balls. In this game, cooperate with your group to keep the balls from falling off the parachute onto the ground. What did you need to do to cooperate to achieve your goal?

Learning Log

My goal this week: _____

_____

		Minutes Read:
Monday	_____ _____ _____ _____	_____
Tuesday	_____ _____ _____ _____	Minutes Read: _____
Wednesday	_____ _____ _____ _____	Minutes Read: _____
Thursday	_____ _____ _____ _____	Minutes Read: _____
Friday	_____ _____ _____ _____	Minutes Read: _____
Home/School Communication		

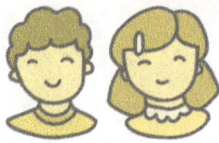

Giving and Accepting Compliments

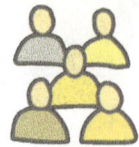

To give people compliments means to say something nice about them. It is a way to help them feel good and confident about themselves. When you give someone a compliment, you need to make eye contact and maintain a friendly face. The compliment you give should be true, specific, and based on the other person's strengths and qualities. For example, while "You're cool" or "I like your shirt" are compliments, they are not specific or based on someone's strengths or qualities. An example of a more specific compliment is, "You worked really hard on that story."

When someone compliments you, it is important to make eye contact and listen to what they are saying. You should accept the compliment, by saying "Thank you," or tell them something about the thing they are complimenting you for. As an example, for the compliment above, you could say, "Thank you. I did work hard on that story. It took me two weeks!"

Practice:

Think of some people you'd like to compliment. It could be a person who works in the lunchroom, someone who plays with you at recess, your teacher, a friend, or someone else. What compliment would you give to that person?

Who?	Compliment

Extension:

As a class, make a paper chain of compliments about each other. Use strips of paper to write compliments about classmates. Staple or tape them into loops on a chain before using them to decorate the classroom. Keep extra strips around so that they can be added to the chain. How does it feel to give a compliment to a classmate? How does it feel to read a compliment that someone has written about you?

Learning Log

My goal this week: _____

_____

Monday	_____ _____ _____ _____	Minutes Read: _____
Tuesday	_____ _____ _____ _____	Minutes Read: _____
Wednesday	_____ _____ _____ _____	Minutes Read: _____
Thursday	_____ _____ _____ _____	Minutes Read: _____
Friday	_____ _____ _____ _____	Minutes Read: _____
Home/School Communication		

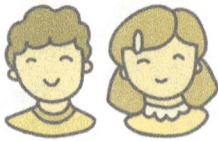

Kindness Challenge

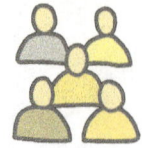

Kindness is treating others in a way that could bring them happiness. In order to be kind, you must treat yourself and others with respect. Being kind to others is like a gift that we can give them. This week, we are going to start a Kindness Challenge. Imagine how much kindness there will be in your school and community if all of you work together to spread kindness—it can be contagious!

Practice:

What does kindness mean to you?

_____

_____

_____

Now, it's time to get to work. Work with your class to make a plan about how you want to spread kindness together. Consider what you will do and how you will keep track of your acts of kindness. Here are some suggestions:

- Make a calendar of kind acts to send home with each student so that they can work on them with their families at home.
- Write thank you notes. How many people can you think of that you'd like to thank? Try to include people that you don't usually say thank you to, such as the bus driver or the person who works in the cafeteria.
- Make posters of ways to be kind to put around the school. The posters could have acts of kindness written on tabs at the bottom that can be ripped off and spread around.
- Set up a compliment corner somewhere in the school where you can encourage students from other classes to write compliments for others and give them to those who they are complimenting.
- Write a kindness pledge and have your whole class sign it and say it every day.
- Plan ways to help others and other acts of service. How many can you do as a class?

After completing the kindness challenge, take some time to talk as a class about how it went. Discuss these questions:

- Was the kindness challenge successful? How do you know?
- Who did the kindness challenge affect?
- What was the most surprising result of the kindness challenge?
- What would you like to continue doing?
- Did your idea of what kindness is change throughout this time?

Learning Log

My goal this week: _____

_____

		Minutes Read:
Monday	_____ _____ _____ _____	_____
Tuesday	_____ _____ _____ _____	Minutes Read: _____
Wednesday	_____ _____ _____ _____	Minutes Read: _____
Thursday	_____ _____ _____ _____	Minutes Read: _____
Friday	_____ _____ _____ _____	Minutes Read: _____
Home/School Communication		

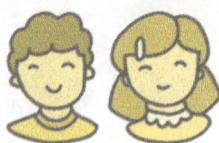

A Place to Belong Review
(Review # 3)

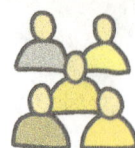

Reflection:

Look over the last nine lessons, from Celebrating Differences to the Kindness Challenge. What is one thing that you've been thinking about and working on lately?

_____

_____

_____

What is something you'd like to start working on?

_____

_____

_____

As a class:

Take some time to do some of the activities written below:

Make a class book celebrating differences that make each student special. Each student can make a page about something that makes them unique and special. For example, "Anette lives with her mom, her aunt, and her grandma" and "Quentin is learning how to tap dance."

Play a game with a parachute and lots of balls. If you don't have a parachute and can't borrow one, you can use a sheet or blanket. In this game, cooperate with your group in order to keep the balls from falling off the parachute onto the ground.

Do a compliment circle. Each student draws the name of another student early in the day and is given some time to think about a compliment for that student. Later, have a compliment circle, where each student compliments the student whose name was drawn and that student accepts the compliment.

Write skits to show ways of resolving conflicts. Act them out for students in a class with younger students.

Write a class story about one or more of the following topics: compromising, apologizing, disagreeing in a respectful way.

Learning Log

My goal this week: _____

_____

Monday	_____ _____ _____ _____	Minutes Read: _____
Tuesday	_____ _____ _____ _____	Minutes Read: _____
Wednesday	_____ _____ _____ _____	Minutes Read: _____
Thursday	_____ _____ _____ _____	Minutes Read: _____
Friday	_____ _____ _____ _____	Minutes Read: _____
Home/School Communication		

Goal Check-In

Look back at the goals you set for yourself at the beginning of the year or the last Goal Check-In. Write the number of two goals here and add notes to check in or make changes to your goals. It's ok to add to or change your goals a little, but keep pushing yourself to grow this year. If you feel you have met your goal, make a new goal for yourself at the bottom of this page.

Goal _____: *Circle one of the options below.*

I've completed this goal!   I'm still working on this goal.   I'm struggling with this goal and need help.

What I need to adjust or continue working on, and who can help me:_____

_____

Goal _____: *Circle one of the options below.*

I've completed this goal!   I'm still working on this goal.   I'm struggling with this goal and need help.

What I need to adjust or continue working on, and who can help me:_____

_____

New goal:

Goal _____: _____

_____

Date you will accomplish this goal: _____

Steps you will take to reach this goal: _____

_____

Who can you ask for help with this goal? _____

How will you know you've accomplished this goal? _____

_____

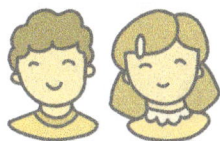

Social-Emotional Learning Connection

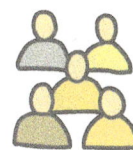

Think about a book you loved reading or listening to lately.

What was the title of the book? _____

What did you love about this book? Draw a picture or write your answer below.

What was one of the big problems or conflicts in this book? How did the characters resolve the conflict? Did any of the characters use a tool we've discussed in our SEL PLanner? How did this tool work for them? Draw or write your answers below.

Notes

Notes

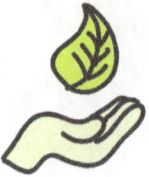

A Healthy Well-being

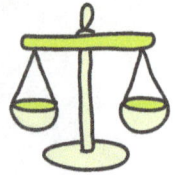

A healthy well-being focuses on all the elements that make you happy. Throughout this theme the social-emotional competencies emphasized are self-management and responsible decision-making.

Throughout this theme, you will be focusing on:
1. Mindfulness (Impulse control, Stress management, & Self-discipline)
2. Being flexible (Identifying problems & Solving problems)
3. Taking Risks (Analyzing situations & Ethical responsibility)
4. Self-esteem and confidence (Self-motivation & Goal-setting)
5. Perseverance (Solving problems, Self-motivation, & Goal-setting)
6. Waiting (Evaluating & Impulse Control)
7. Being a role model (Self-discipline)
8. Gratitude (Ethical responsibility)

Caring for yourself and ensuring you are healthy on the inside and the outside is important to your overall well-being. The books on the list below emphasize how you can care for yourself inside and out!

Abracadabra! The Magic of Trying by Maria Loretta Giraldo
I am Peace: a book of Mindfulness by Susan Verde
Puppy Mind by Andrew Jordan Nance and Jim Durk
Lemonade Hurricane by Licia Morelli
Charlotte and the Quiet Place by Deborah Sosin
Quiet by Tomie dePaola
Listening to my Body by Gabi Garcia
Breathe Like a Bear by Kira Willey
My Magic Breath by Nick Ortner
Have You Filled a Bucket Today? By Carol McCloud
The Hugging Tree by Jill Neimark
My Heart by Corinna Luyken
Emmanuel's Dream by Laurie Ann Thompson
What Should Danny Do? By Adir Levy and Granit Levy

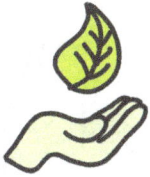

A Healthy Well-being

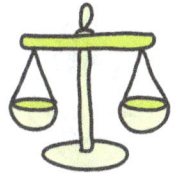

Well-being is about being healthy on the inside and outside. Draw a picture (and write a few words in your picture) that show what you do to stay healthy in your life.

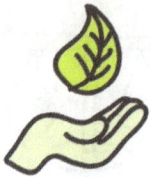

Mindfulness

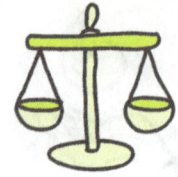

Mindfulness is a way of slowing down and focusing your attention. It allows you to notice your emotions, how your body feels, and what your mind is doing. It can be a helpful way to feel relaxed and calm.

Think back to when you learned to do belly breathing and bunny breathing. Today, you are going to learn another way to help you focus on your breathing. First, sit with your feet on the floor and close your eyes. Count to 10 for each breath in this way:

Breathe in = 1	Breathe out = 6
Breathe out = 2	Breathe in = 7
Breathe in = 3	Breathe out = 8
Breathe out = 4	Breathe in = 9
Breathe in = 5	Breathe out = 10

Then, start over. If you find that you've lost focus and are at number 12, start back at one again.

Practice:
Try to do some mindfulness techniques (belly breathing, bunny breathing, breathing counting to 10, etc.) three times this week. Circle how you feel before and after.

Day	Before				After			
	Angry	Scared	Nervous	Sad	Angry	Scared	Nervous	Sad
	Excited	Frustrated	Happy	Calm	Excited	Frustrated	Happy	Calm
	Angry	Scared	Nervous	Sad	Angry	Scared	Nervous	Sad
	Excited	Frustrated	Happy	Calm	Excited	Frustrated	Happy	Calm
	Angry	Scared	Nervous	Sad	Angry	Scared	Nervous	Sad
	Excited	Frustrated	Happy	Calm	Excited	Frustrated	Happy	Calm

Extension:
Do a mindful eating activity. Use a small piece of chocolate or a raisin.
Notice what it looks like, smells like, sounds like, and feels like. What did you notice while eating that you haven't noticed before? When do you think you might use this activity again?

Learning Log

My goal this week: _____

_____

		Minutes Read:
Monday	_____ _____ _____ _____	_____
Tuesday	_____ _____ _____ _____	Minutes Read: _____
Wednesday	_____ _____ _____ _____	Minutes Read: _____
Thursday	_____ _____ _____ _____	Minutes Read: _____
Friday	_____ _____ _____ _____	Minutes Read: _____
Home/School Communication		

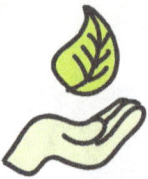

Being Flexible

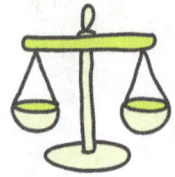

Sometimes, when you are playing or working with someone, you may want one thing but the other person wants something else. We have already learned how to compromise, but there are times when it makes more sense to be flexible and let the other person have their way. In order to find out when is a good time to be flexible, think about how your actions affect others. For example, if you always sit in the chair next to the teacher, but your friend really wants to sit in that chair today, think about how you can solve that problem. You can think about how your friend would feel if you sat in that chair and also how your friend would feel if you let them sit in that chair today. You can also think about how much of a big deal it would be to you if you sat in another chair. Use that information to help you decide if you can be flexible and sit somewhere else today, or if you need to work out a compromise. Usually, when something is not really important to you, but it is a big deal to someone else, you can be flexible.

Practice:
Circle flexible or compromise based on what you would do in these situations.

Your sister wants to hang her backpack on the hook that you usually hang your jacket on, even though there are two other empty hooks.

Flexible / Compromise

Usually, you read first when you do partner reading, but today, your partner wants to read first.

Flexible / Compromise

At recess, you and a friend really want to play soccer, but your other friends really want to play kickball.

Flexible / Compromise

You like to be the first in line to go to lunch, but another student got there before you today.

Flexible / Compromise

Only one rainbow pencil is left in the pencil box today. You really want to use it, but so do all of the other students at your table.

Flexible / Compromise

Your teacher gives you a partner to work with during math time, but you want to work with your best friend.

Flexible / Compromise

Extension:
Use puppets to act out situations where you can be flexible. If you'd like, you can use some of the situations from above. Afterwards, talk to a partner about how you can tell the difference between a time when it makes sense to be flexible and a time when it makes sense to compromise.

Learning Log

My goal this week: _____

_____

Monday	_____ _____ _____ _____	Minutes Read: _____
Tuesday	_____ _____ _____ _____	Minutes Read: _____
Wednesday	_____ _____ _____ _____	Minutes Read: _____
Thursday	_____ _____ _____ _____	Minutes Read: _____
Friday	_____ _____ _____ _____	Minutes Read: _____
Home/School Communication		

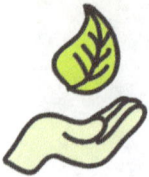

Self-esteem and Confidence

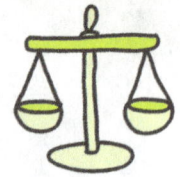

To have self-esteem is to believe in yourself and be proud of what you can do. It is similar to being confident, which we talked about when we talked about emotions. You can build your self-esteem and confidence in many ways. Some of them are:

- Think about things that you are good at
- Use positive self-talk
- Keep track of your successes
- Set and achieve realistic goals
- Try again when you haven't been successful

Practice:

Use this space to draw, make a collage, or use words to represent everything that you can do that makes you confident and proud of who you are.

Extension:

Think back to the lesson about self-talk. Discuss with a partner as to how you can use self-talk to build your confidence and self-esteem. What would you say to yourself in a situation in which you need to build confidence? How would that help you?

Learning Log

My goal this week: _____

_____

		Minutes Read:
Monday	_____ _____ _____ _____	_____
Tuesday	_____ _____ _____ _____	Minutes Read: _____
Wednesday	_____ _____ _____ _____	Minutes Read: _____
Thursday	_____ _____ _____ _____	Minutes Read: _____
Friday	_____ _____ _____ _____	Minutes Read: _____
Home/School Communication		

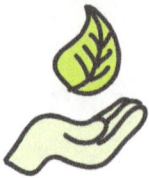

Making Mistakes

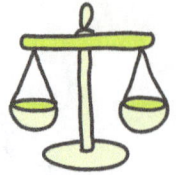

Everyone makes mistakes sometimes, but did you know that mistakes can help us learn? Mistakes can be very important because they can tell us where we need to focus our practice. There are different kinds of mistakes. We want to try to avoid making the kind of mistakes that happen because we weren't paying attention or we were just being careless. But there are other mistakes, which happen because we were trying to do something that was hard for us, that can help us to learn. When we make a mistake, we must ask ourselves this question: "What can I learn from this?" Then, we need to make a plan to try again. It is very important to not be afraid of making mistakes because if you don't make mistakes, then you can't learn from them.

Practice:

Try to do something that is difficult for you here. Solve a hard math problem, spell a hard word, draw something that is hard for you to draw, write a poem, etc. Use a pen or marker.	Now, look back at what you worked on in the other box to see if you made any mistakes. Use a pencil here and try to do it again, in order to learn from the mistakes that you made.

Extension:

Learn about some mistakes that became successes. Do some research to find out more about them or read some books. Possible books to check out:

- *Mistakes that Worked: 40 Familiar Inventions & How They Came to Be* by Charlotte Foltz Jones
- *Famous Fails!: Mighty Mistakes, Mega Mishaps, & How a Mess Can Lead to Success!* by Crispin Boyer

After learning about them, speak to a classmate about how you can turn your own mistakes into successes and a learning experience.

Learning Log

My goal this week: _____

_____

		Minutes Read:
Monday	_____ _____ _____ _____	____
Tuesday	_____ _____ _____ _____	____
Wednesday	_____ _____ _____ _____	____
Thursday	_____ _____ _____ _____	____
Friday	_____ _____ _____ _____	____
Home/School Communication		

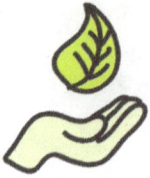

Trying New Things

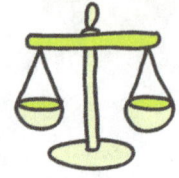

Sometimes, it can feel a little bit scary to try new things, but it is important to try new things because we can learn from them. Trying something new can mean taking a risk or the possibility of making a mistake. In such situations, we have to use positive self-talk and tell ourselves we can do it, and then try our best.

When something new seems overwhelming, one thing you can do is to take small steps that will help you get there eventually. For example, if singing on stage for the class performance seems like a very hard task, then break it down into smaller steps. First, try singing at home in front of the mirror. Then, sing in front of your family. Next, sing in front of a group of friends. Then, try singing on the stage with your class. You'll build confidence each time, which means that you'll be ready when it's time to sing for the performance.

Another tool you can use to try new things is to practice something new before you have to do it. For example, if you feel unsure about going to the dentist, then talk about what you'll do there and practice what will happen at home with your family.

Practice:
Think about a time when you tried something new. How did you feel before you did it?

_____

_____

_____

Did you do anything that made it easier for you? How did you feel after you did it?

_____

_____

_____

Extension:
Create a "Challenge Journal" for yourself (we've made one for you on the next page to get you started). Each time you are brave and try something new, write about it in your journal. Write about how you felt before you did it, what you did to help you try that new thing, and how you felt after you did it.

Learning Log

My goal this week: _____

_____

		Minutes Read:
Monday	_____ _____ _____ _____	_____
Tuesday	_____ _____ _____ _____	Minutes Read: _____
Wednesday	_____ _____ _____ _____	Minutes Read: _____
Thursday	_____ _____ _____ _____	Minutes Read: _____
Friday	_____ _____ _____ _____	Minutes Read: _____
Home/School Communication		

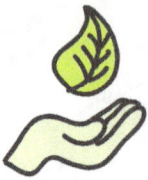

Challenge Journal

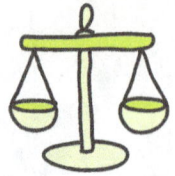

In our lesson Trying New Things, we talked about creating a Challenge Journal. Use this space as your Challenge Journal. Each time you are brave and try something new, write about it in your journal. Write about how you felt before you did it, what you did to help you try that new thing, and how you felt after you did it.

A time I was brave and tried something new was...

Before I did this, I felt...	What I did to help me try this new thing:

How I felt after I did it!

A time I was brave and tried something new was...

Before I did this, I felt...	What I did to help me try this new thing:

How I felt after I did it!

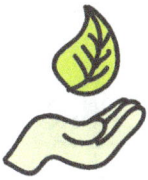

Challenge Journal

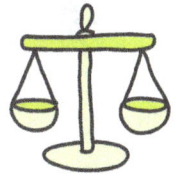

A time I was brave and tried something new was...

Before I did this, I felt...

What I did to help me try this new thing:

How I felt after I did it!

A time I was brave and tried something new was...

Before I did this, I felt...

What I did to help me try this new thing:

How I felt after I did it!

Continue your Challenge Journal on your own using a notebook or the notes pages in this planner.

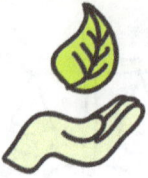

COLORING PAGE

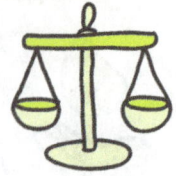

These stars can be used to help you breathe mindfully. Use your crayon or pencil and start by going UP one of the points while you breathe in, then trace going down the point of the star and breathe out. Continue this four more times until you get around all five points of the star. Then try this breathing exercise for a different sized star on the page.

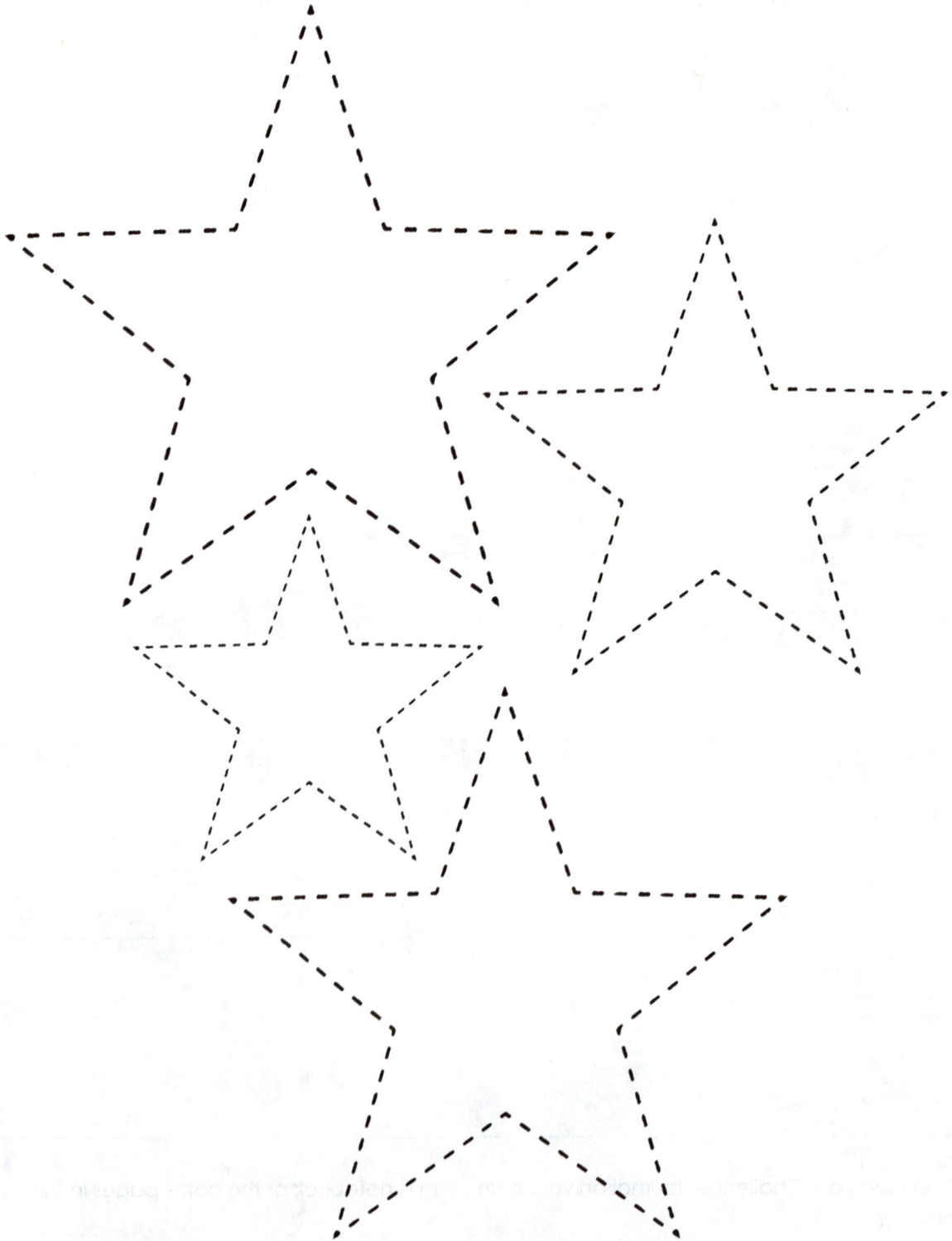

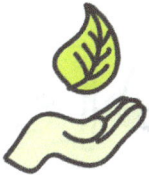

COLORING PAGE

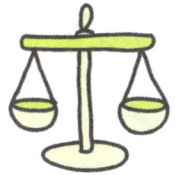

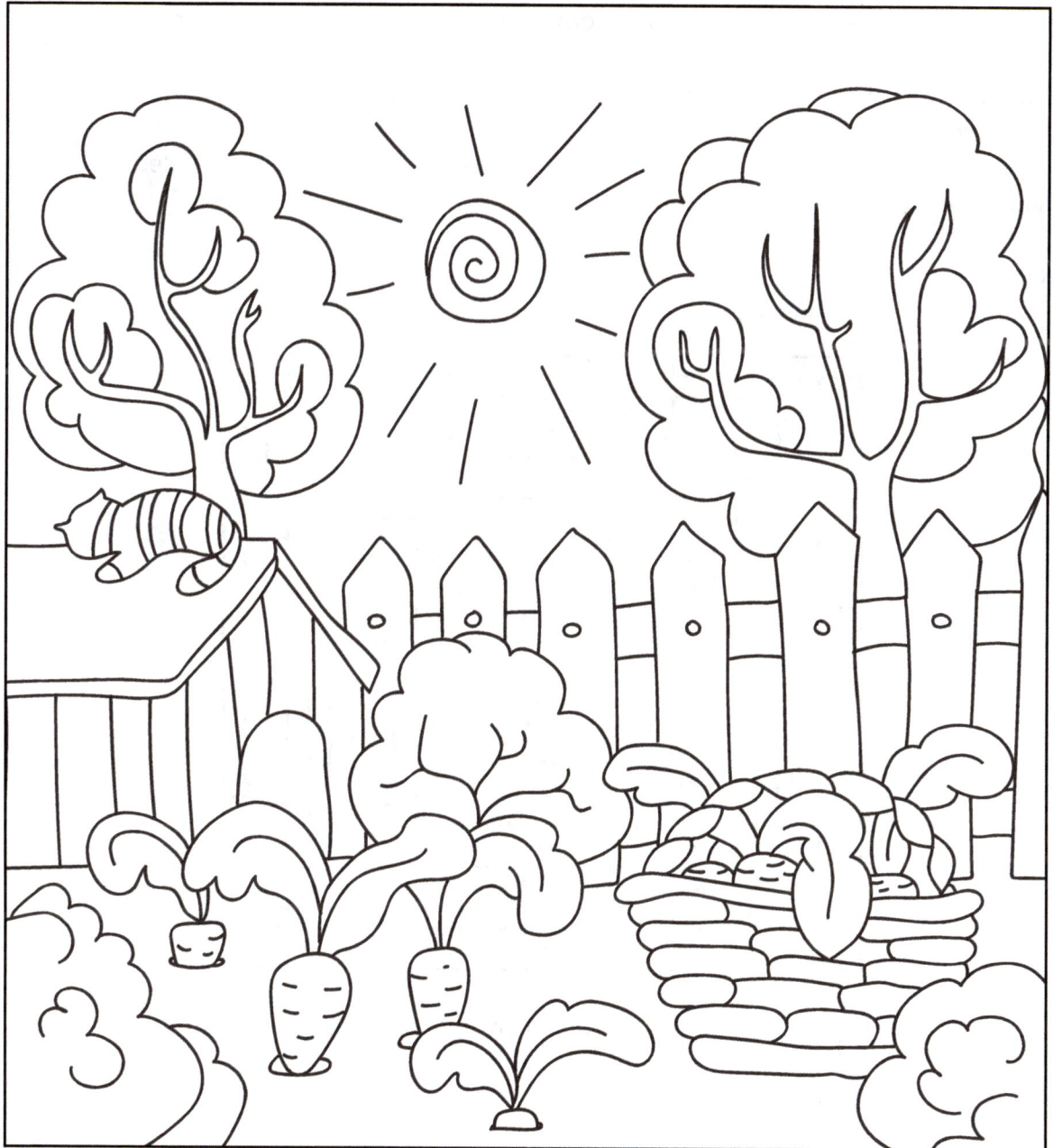

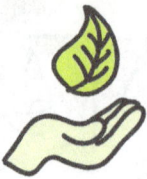

Perseverance

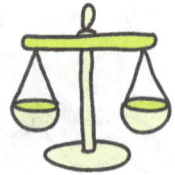

Perseverance is what helps someone keep trying to do something even if it is difficult. It is an important quality because it helps us to move past things that are hard and onto the things that we want to achieve. In order to have perseverance, we need to use both our ability and our self-control. We might struggle to do something hard, but this struggle helps us to grow. Like we talked about a couple of weeks ago, mistakes give us the chance to persevere. We might not be able to do something yet, but practice leads to progress.

When we are struggling with something and need to persevere, one thing we can do is to stop and take a break. We can then think about what is working and what is not, which can help us continue doing the things that are working. Along the way, we can celebrate small successes we have as we continue to persevere until we complete the task.

Practice:

Try completing the maze below.

How did you use perseverance as you worked on the maze? How did it feel?

_____

_____

_____

Extension:

Read or retell The Tortoise and the Hare. How did the tortoise show perseverance? Did he use any other skills that you've learned about?

Learning Log

My goal this week: _____

_____

		Minutes Read:
Monday	_____ _____ _____ _____	_____
Tuesday	_____ _____ _____ _____	Minutes Read: _____
Wednesday	_____ _____ _____ _____	Minutes Read: _____
Thursday	_____ _____ _____ _____	Minutes Read: _____
Friday	_____ _____ _____ _____	Minutes Read: _____
Home/School Communication		

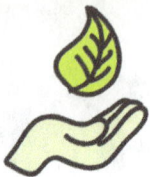

Waiting Patiently

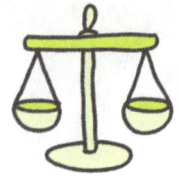

There are times in life when you need to wait patiently. Being patient means that you stay calm while you wait. For example, you may need to wait patiently when you are in a restaurant, on a car or bus ride, or while your friends are having a turn with a toy that you'd like to use. When you wait, there are things that you can do to make the waiting easier for you. You can use your imagination, sing a song, play a game, or find another way to keep yourself busy.

Practice:
Choose a way to wait patiently for each example of a time when you'd need to wait.

1. _____ Your mom is talking on the phone.   a. Use your imagination to make up a story.

2. _____ You finish your math test early.   b. Play 20 questions with someone.

3. _____ You are waiting in the waiting room   c. Add details to your writing or drawing.
before your doctor's appointment.

4. _____ You need the red marker to finish   d. Read a book to yourself.
your drawing, but your friend is using it now.

5. _____ You finished your writing and want   e. Draw a picture.
to show it to your teacher, but she is working
with another student.

6. _____ You ordered your food at a restau-   f. Count as high as you can. Then skip count
rant and are waiting for it to come.   by 10s, 5s, and 2s.

7. _____ You are on a long car/bus ride.   g. Sing a song to yourself.

Extension:
Talk to a partner about a time when you needed to wait patiently. What did you do as you waited? Were you able to wait patiently for as long as you needed to? Work together to make a list of things that you can do when you have to wait patiently.

Learning Log

My goal this week: _____

_____

		Minutes Read:
Monday	_____ _____ _____ _____	_____
Tuesday	_____ _____ _____ _____	_____
Wednesday	_____ _____ _____ _____	_____
Thursday	_____ _____ _____ _____	_____
Friday	_____ _____ _____ _____	_____
Home/School Communication		

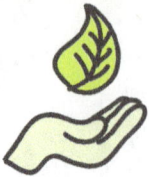

Being a Role Model

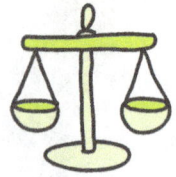

Role models are people who you look up to and admire. They make others want to be like them by being examples and without directly teaching how to be like them. If they are positive role models, then they can inspire positive actions in others.

If you want to be a role model, pay attention to your words and actions. For example, you should do the things that you say you are going to do. You should act in kind and respectful ways. You also must use kind and respectful words. If someone is looking up to you, then you need to act in a way that you'd like someone to imitate.

Practice:
Think about people in your life who you look up to as role models. What things do you admire about them? In what ways do they act like role models?

Person	Things you admire	Ways they act like role models

What can you do to make sure that you are a role model for others?

_____

_____

_____

Extension:
Write a letter to one of the role models that you chose above. Tell that person why they are a role model to you and how it makes you feel. Include a plan for ways in which you can be a role model for others.

Learning Log

My goal this week: _____

_____

Monday	_____ _____ _____ _____	Minutes Read: _____
Tuesday	_____ _____ _____ _____	Minutes Read: _____
Wednesday	_____ _____ _____ _____	Minutes Read: _____
Thursday	_____ _____ _____ _____	Minutes Read: _____
Friday	_____ _____ _____ _____	Minutes Read: _____
Home/School Communication		

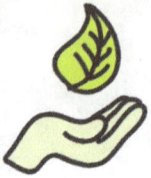

Gratitude

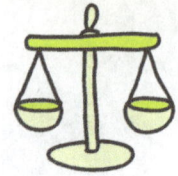

The word gratitude is related to the word grateful, which means thankful. Taking time to think about what you're grateful for can help you to develop an attitude of gratitude. By doing so, you can notice the positive things that are happening around you and be thankful for them.

There are many ways in which you can show gratitude. One very basic way is to say thank you. Another is to notice all of the wonderful things that are happening around you. You can also show gratitude by helping others, volunteering, and giving to others.

Practice:
Use this space to draw, make a collage, or use words to represent the things for which you are grateful.

Extension:
Make a space in the classroom for gratitude. Here are some possibilities:
- A gratitude jar, where students write down the things that they are grateful for on small strips of paper and put them in the jar.
- A gratitude tree, where students write down the things that they are grateful for on leaves and add them to the tree.
- A class gratitude journal, where students write down the things that they are grateful for.
- A class gratitude bulletin board, where students can add the things that they are grateful for at any time.

Every once in a while, take some time to read through and think about some of the things that students are thankful for.

Learning Log

My goal this week: _____

_____

		Minutes Read:
Monday	_____ _____ _____ _____	Minutes Read: _____
Tuesday	_____ _____ _____ _____	Minutes Read: _____
Wednesday	_____ _____ _____ _____	Minutes Read: _____
Thursday	_____ _____ _____ _____	Minutes Read: _____
Friday	_____ _____ _____ _____	Minutes Read: _____
Home/School Communication		

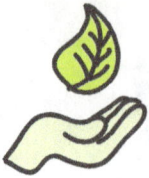

A Healthy Wellbeing Review
(Review # 4)

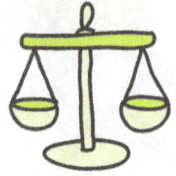

Reflection:

Look over the last nine lessons, from Mindfulness to Gratitude. What is one thing that you've been thinking about and working on lately?

_____

_____

_____

What is something you'd like to start working on?

_____

_____

_____

As a class:

Take some time to do some of these activities:

Spend some time each day doing mindfulness activities. Practice the breathing exercises that you've learned or look for a guided mindfulness activity in a book or on YouTube. In the classroom, talk to your classmates about how mindfulness affects the way students are feeling and when students think are the best times of the day to incorporate mindfulness activities.

Make an "I can" list, book, or jar. Every time you try something new, write down what you can do. For example, "I can write my last name." or "I can cross the monkey bars."

Work on some difficult puzzles or mazes to build perseverance.

Write thank you notes to people around the school to show you are thankful for the things they do.

Play a game like Memory to practice waiting patiently for your turn.

Write skits to show ways of being a role model. Act them out for students in a class with younger students.

Learning Log

My goal this week: _____

_____

		Minutes Read:
Monday	_____ _____ _____ _____	_____
Tuesday	_____ _____ _____ _____	_____
Wednesday	_____ _____ _____ _____	_____
Thursday	_____ _____ _____ _____	_____
Friday	_____ _____ _____ _____	_____
Home/School Communication		

Goal Check-In

Look back at the goals you set for yourself at the beginning of the year or the last Goal Check-In. Write the number of two goals here and add notes to check in or make changes to your goals. It's ok to add to or change your goals a little, but keep pushing yourself to grow this year. If you feel you have met your goal, make a new goal for yourself at the bottom of this page.

Goal _____: *Circle one of the options below.*

I've completed this goal!   I'm still working on this goal.   I'm struggling with this goal
                                                                             and need help.

What I need to adjust or continue working on, and who can help me:_____

_____

Goal _____: *Circle one of the options below.*

I've completed this goal!   I'm still working on this goal.   I'm struggling with this goal
                                                                             and need help.

What I need to adjust or continue working on, and who can help me:_____

_____

New goal:

Goal _____: _____

_____

Date you will accomplish this goal: _____

Steps you will take to reach this goal: _____

_____

Who can you ask for help with this goal? _____

How will you know you've accomplished this goal? _____

_____

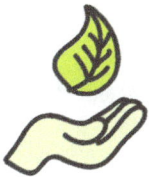

Social-Emotional Learning Connection

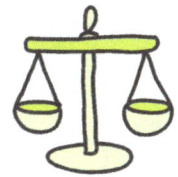

Think about a book you loved reading or listening to lately.

What was the title of the book? _____

What did you love about this book? Draw a picture or write your answer below.

What happened when or if the character, or characters, made a mistake? Did they use any of the tools we've learned about in our SEL planner to help them? What tools did they use? Draw or write your answers below.

Notes

Reflect on Your Goals

You can find your goals on pages 8-9.

Goal #1: _____

_____

How did it go? _____

_____

Goal #2: _____

_____

How did it go? _____

_____

Goal #3: _____

_____

How did it go? _____

_____

What is one goal that you have for the summer or next school year?

Goal: _____

_____

Date you will accomplish this goal: _____

Steps you will take to reach this goal:

1. _____

2. _____

3. _____

Who can you ask for help with this goal? _____

How will you know you've accomplished this goal? _____

_____

Books I Read This Year

Track the books you have read this school year on the chart below.

Title	Author	My thoughts on this book

Transitioning to summer

The school year is coming to an end, so it will soon be summer break. Summer break can be different for different people—for some kids, it means going to summer school or day camp all day everyday. For others, it means a lot of open-ended free time. Think about what summer break is going to be like for you. If you're not sure, ask your parent or carer to tell you more about what you'll be doing during the summer break.

Sometimes, change can be difficult. When one thing ends and another begins, it can be hard to adjust to the new routines. Some things that can help you adjust to the changes are to ask questions about what will be happening so you know what to expect, talk to others about how you're feeling, and to write or draw about your feelings.

As you go into the summer, remember that you learned so many new skills and you have so many tools that you can use to help you in all kinds of different situations. You can look back through this planner to remind you of how to use these skills anytime you need to!

How are you feeling about the end of the school year and the beginning of summer break? Why do you feel that way?

_____

_____

_____

Draw and/or write in the boxes below.

What is something you'll miss from school while you're away this summer?	What is something you're looking forward to this summer?

Summer challenge: Try to challenge yourself to incorporate one of the practices you learned this school year into your daily life. Maybe you'll try to do an act of kindness each day or you'll do some mindfulness techniques daily or you'll start a daily gratitude practice. What can you challenge yourself to do?

Read a book this summer!
Kindergarten

Here are some can't-put-down summer reads. Use the chart to select the best book for you (and remember you can find these books at your school or community library, so you don't have to buy the book to read it!).

What kind of book do you want to read?

Wordless picture book

Travel to another world

OR

Laugh out loud

What would you do if you met another you?

Will baby bird learn how to fly?

Read: *Another* by Christian Robinson

Read: *Fly!!* by Mark Teague

Book to read by myself

Scared and Silly

OR

Sweet & Heart-warming?

Duck is scared... but who he is scared of will make you laugh!

A prickly porcupine wants a hug!

Read: *What is Chasing Duck* by Jan Thomas

Read: *I Need a Hug* by Aaron Blabey

Love to read?

Read all four books! You can find more book recommendations from your Librarian or on readbrightly.com

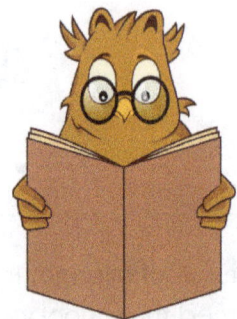

Read a book this summer!

1st Grade

What kind of book do you want to read?

Book about an animal

Tortoise

OR

Ducks & Porcupines

Truman is tired of waiting. Will he find his best friend again?

Read: *Truman* by Jean Reidy

Big Duck, Little Duck, and Porcupine love to explore and be creative

Read: *Duck, Duck, Porcupine* by Salina Yoon

Book about a journey

Math

OR

Nature

Triangle is going to play a trick on his friends! Find out how!

Read: *Triangle* by Jon Klassen

Three girls go on an afternoon hike. What will they see, hear, and do?

Read: *The hike* by Alison Farrell

Love to read?

Read all four books! You can find more book recommendations from your Librarian or on readbrightly.com

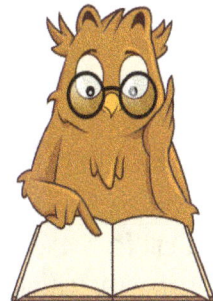

Read a book this summer!

2nd Grade

What kind of book do you wanna read?

Fiction

Confident girl OR **Magical Creatures**

Yasmin is a 2nd grader with a BIG imagination!

Would you want a magical creature as your PET?

Read: *Meet Yasmin! By Saadia Faruqui*

Read: *Miss Turie's Magic Creatures by Joy Keller*

Nonfiction

Science OR **Nature**

Meet biologist Ernest Everett Just who observes sea creatures and makes big discoveries!

Enjoy a book of poetry about the changing of seasons.

Read: *The Vast Wonder of the World by Mélin Mangal*

Read: *When Green Becomes Tomatoes by Julie Fogliano*

Love to read?

Read all four books! You can find more book recommendations from your Librarian or on readbrightly.com

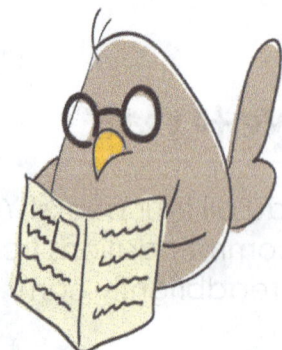

Top 10 Habits of Social-Emotional Learning

1. Journal about my thoughts and feelings.

2. Breathe mindfully.

3. Identify my emotions and tell others how I feel.

4. Practice a growth mindset.

5. Ask for help from a trusted adult when I need it.

6. Create goals that I can accomplish within a certain time period.

7. Read books from different perspectives and different places.

8. Make new friends and include others in my group of friends.

9. Be kind.

10. Disagree respectfully.

Ways to be Mindful

Belly Breathing

Lay on the floor with a small stuffed animal on your belly (not your chest). As you breathe in deeply through your nose and out through your mouth, feel your stuffy rise slowly and come back down. Slowly rock your stuffy to sleep with your belly breaths.

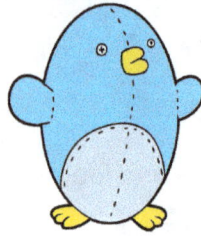

Partner Breathing

Sit on the floor back to back with a friend. Focus first on your breath for 3 slow inhales. Then bring your attention to feeling your partner breathe. Slowly start to sync up your breaths so that you are both breathing in and out together.

Bunny Breathing

Sit on your knees. Take three quick breaths in through your nose, like a bunny sniffing. Breathe out slowly through your mouth. Repeat.

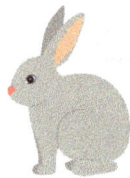

Counting to 10

First, sit with your feet on the floor and close your eyes. Count to 10 for each breath in this way:

Breathe in = 1
Breathe out = 2
Breathe in = 3
Breathe out = 4
Breathe in = 5
Breathe out = 6
Breathe in = 7
Breathe out = 8
Breathe in = 9
Breathe out = 10

Then, start over. If you find that you've lost focus and are at number 12, start back at one again.

Teamwork Soup

As a class, work together with your teacher to fill out your teamwork soup chart. What do we all need to bring to be a kind and compassionate class who works together and supports one another? Use the carrots example, then add in your thoughts to make the soup delicious for all.

Ingredients	What is the ingredient a symbol for? Why do we need it?	Who needs to bring it?
Carrots	They are a symbol of **creativity** because they are bright in color and snappy when you break and share them.	Everyone

When you are in class, working in groups, and even out on the playground, remember to bring your teamwork soup ingredients!

Dictionary of Emotions

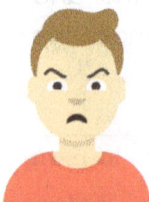

ANGRY

When you feel mad.

<u>What to do:</u> First, take a deep breath or take a minute to be quiet and collect your thoughts. When you feel calmer, you can explain how you are feeling, what is making you feel that way, and look for a solution. Some things you can do when you are feeling angry are drawing, writing, moving your body (running, playing a sport, etc.), spending some time alone, and meditation.

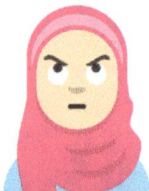

FRUSTRATED

When you feel angry or unhappy because you are trying to do something, but are not being successful.

<u>What to do:</u> First, take a break from what you are doing. Try taking a deep breath or taking a minute to be quiet and think about the best thing to do next. When you feel calmer, you can explain to someone else what you are trying to do and ask for help.

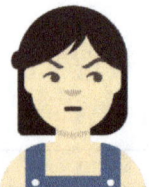

JEALOUS

When you feel unhappy or angry because someone else has something that you want or is doing something that you want to do.

<u>What to do:</u> Talk to someone about how you are feeling. Think about the people and things in your life that you are grateful for. If there is a way to change the situation you are feeling jealous about, work on making that change.

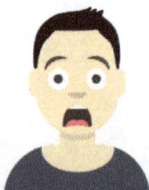

SCARED

When you feel afraid.

<u>What to do:</u> Talk to someone about why you are scared. Try to take small steps toward doing things that you feel scared of with someone you trust.

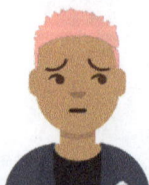

NERVOUS

When you feel worried or afraid of what might happen.

<u>What to do:</u> Tell someone what you are feeling, so they can understand and try to help. Talk to them about what might happen. Ask questions. Make a plan for what you can do. When you feel nervous, it is helpful to take deep breaths to help feel calmer.

Dictionary of Emotions

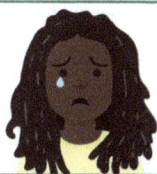

SAD

When you feel unhappy.

<u>What to do:</u> Talk to someone about how you feel. It's OK to cry. Spend time with people who make you feel safe and find things you enjoy doing.

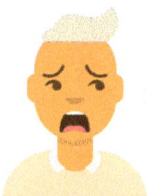

DISAPPOINTED

When you feel unhappy because something you hoped for did not happen.

<u>What to do:</u> Tell someone how you are feeling. Think about what you could do instead. Is there anything good that can come from this situation?

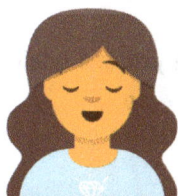

PROUD

When you feel happy because you did something well.

<u>What to do:</u> Congratulate yourself for a job well done. Share your pride with a carer like your mom or a teacher; they will be proud of you! When you feel pride, be careful not to put down others who may not find it as easy to do.

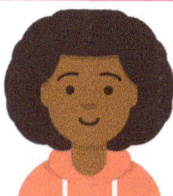

HAPPY

When you feel joy.

<u>What to do:</u> Enjoy this feeling. Try to share your happiness with others by playing with them, sharing with them, or being extra kind.

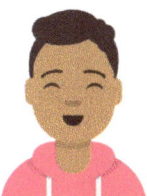

EXCITED

When you feel excited or enthusiastic.

<u>What to do:</u> Laugh, smile, and share your excitement with others. Sometimes, when we feel excited, we are in a place where we need to be calm or quiet, though, and this can be hard since excited can be a louder emotion. If you need to, calm your body by breathing deeply.

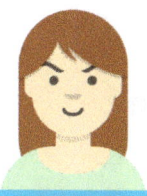

CONFIDENT

When you believe you can do something well.

<u>What to do:</u> Remember how being confident feels in your body because there will be times when you do something and don't feel confident. Consider how you could build confidence when you are working on, or doing something where you don't feel confident.

The Peace Path

Finish the sentences below when having a disagreement. It will help you be heard, solve the problem, and move forward!

Walk the Peace Path

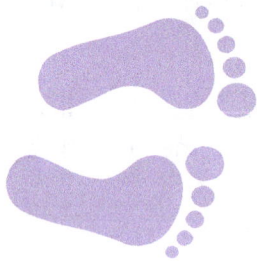 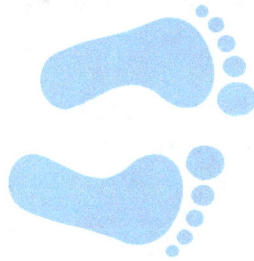 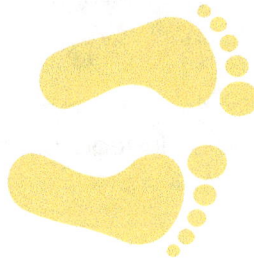 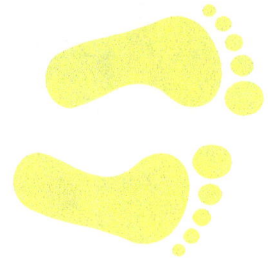

I feel...   **When...**   **I need...**   **Would you be willing to...**

Example: I feel frustrated when you tell me how to color my art project. I need space apart. Would you be willing to let me color by myself for a while?

You try: Think of a time when you and a friend were disagreeing. Use the peace path to solve the problem below.

I feel _____ when _____.

I need

to eat/drink	to rest	bubble space	to feel safe
a trusting friendship	space apart	to play something else	time alone
to try again	someone to talk to	Other: _____	

Would you be willing to_____?

Social-Emotional Learning Stories

Sofia's Story

Sofia is playing freeze tag with a group of friends on the playground. You have been walking around trying to decide what you want to play. You finally decide you want to play freeze tag, so you go over to ask Sofia if you can play. Sofia doesn't answer you; instead, she runs away from you and keeps playing.

What would you do?

Resolution:

You feel sad that Sofia is ignoring you and not letting you play. You realize that you need to get her to stop running so you can talk to her to solve the problem. You walk over to where she is and say, "Sofia, please stop running. I want to talk to you." She's still running, but then she notices that your face looks sad, so she stops. You tell her, "Sofia, I didn't like it when you ran away from me when I was trying to ask you if I could play with you." Sofia repeats back what she heard you say and explains that she was involved in the game and didn't want to stop. She apologizes and asks if you're ready to play now. You say, "Yes!" and then you're both off and running in the game of freeze tag.

Social-Emotional Learning Stories

Read the stories and notice how other kids found solutions using social-emotional learning tools.

Saul's Story

In your class, there is one student named Saul, who is very shy and prefers to stay quiet most of the time. He sits at the end of the table at lunch, so he doesn't have to sit next to anyone else. You've asked him to sit next to you before, but he politely says no, and he seems content to sit by himself. One day, you notice that Julisa, another student in your class, walked past Saul, and took the apple off of his tray. Saul doesn't seem to care, so you don't do anything. The next day, you see that Julisa takes the cookie off of Saul's tray.

What would you do if you saw this?

Resolution:

You know that what you saw was unfair and unkind. The first time you saw it, you didn't do something, but now you see it again, and you know you have to speak up. You walk over to Julisa and say, "That's not your cookie. Give it back." She looks embarrassed that you saw her take it from Saul. She trudges back toward Saul and gives the cookie back. Julisa turns around and sees that you're still standing there looking at her. She asks you what you want. You tell her that what she did was unkind, and she should find a way to fix it. She looks at Saul and apologizes. She tells him that she won't do it again and asks what she can do to make it better. Saul says he forgives her, but he'd prefer to be left alone during lunchtime.

Social-Emotional Learning Checklist

- ☐ I can identify my emotions.
- ☐ I know my strengths.
- ☐ I am confident in myself and can use positive self-talk.

- ☐ I know how to motivate myself to do well, even when things are difficult.
- ☐ I create goals for myself and can achieve them.
- ☐ I manage my stress using breathing or other mindfulness techniques.
- ☐ I can regulate my emotions so I don't hurt others or myself.

- ☐ I understand people have different perspectives and opinions.
- ☐ I am practicing empathy by trying to understand other people's feelings.
- ☐ I read books from different perspectives and keep an open mind.
- ☐ I respect all people and like including new people in my group of friends.

- ☐ I am a good listener.
- ☐ I cooperate well with others and work well in groups.
- ☐ I am confident in who I am and resist peer pressure.
- ☐ I ask for help when I need it.

- ☐ I can identify problems and solve them using a variety of techniques.
- ☐ I reflect on my own well-being and make decisions that are healthy for my body and mind.
- ☐ I try to make choices that are ethical and do not harm people, the environment, or animals.

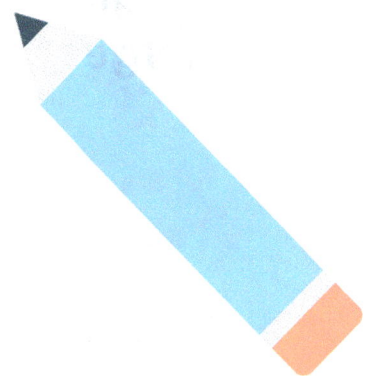

Self-Talk Affirmations

I love **myself**

I am a **reader**

I am a **scientist**

I am **bold**

I am **special**

I am a **mathematician**

I am **strong**

I am **brave**

I am a **writer**

I can **do this**

I can **persevere**

I can **calm myself** down

I am **adventurous**

I can **take charge**

I can **listen carefully**

I can **ask for help**

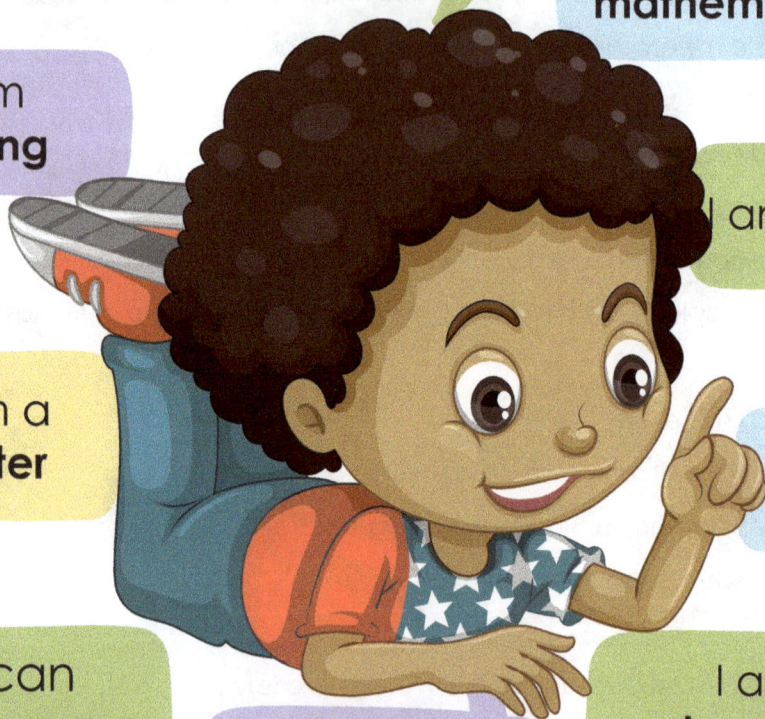

Self-Talk Affirmations

I am **kind**

I am **loved**

I can be a **leader**

I can **help**

I can **say no**

I can make a **difference**

I am **thankful**

I can get **better**

I am a **good friend**

It is **OK** to **feel this way**

I can be **flexible**

I can **resolve** this conflict

I will **be OK**

It is **OK** to **make mistakes**

I have something **to say**

I can **try** new things

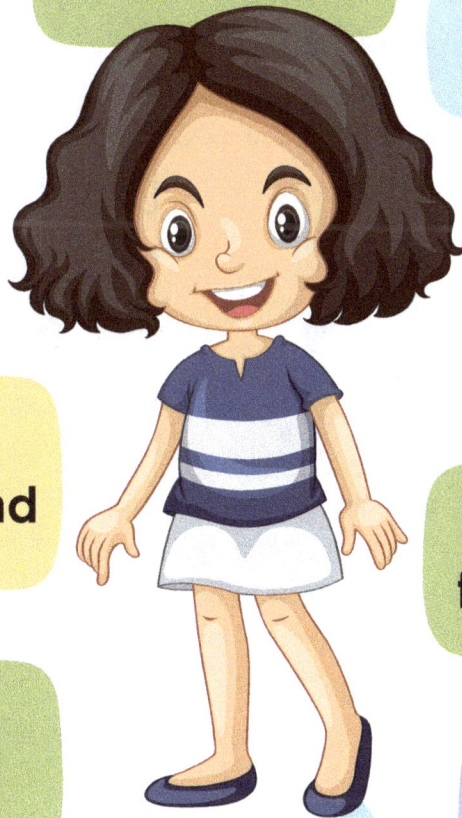

All the Planners in the series:

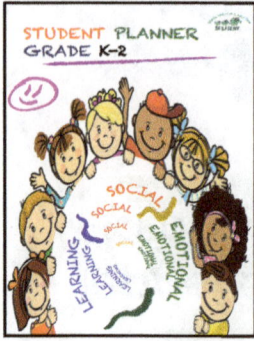

Social Emotional Learning
(SEL) Student Planner
Grades K-2
ISBN: 978-1-7336417-0-8

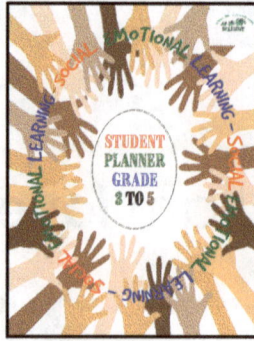

Social Emotional Learning
(SEL) Student Planner
Grades 3-5
ISBN: 978-1-7336417-1-5

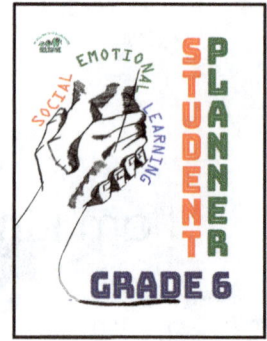

Social Emotional Learning
(SEL) Student Planner
Grade 6
ISBN: 978-1-7336417-2-2

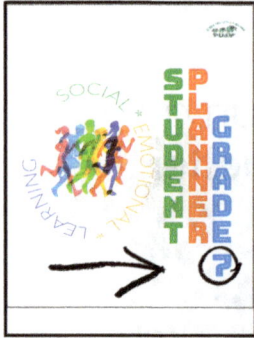

Social Emotional Learning
(SEL) Student Planner
Grade 7
ISBN: 978-1-7336417-3-9

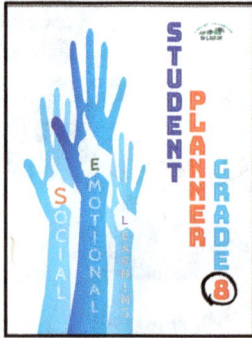

Social Emotional Learning
(SEL) Student Planner
Grade 8
ISBN: 978-1-7336417-7-7

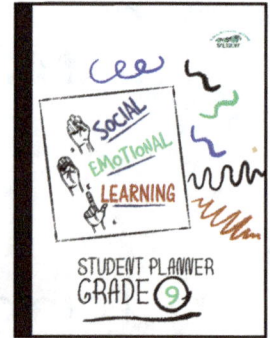

Social Emotional Learning
(SEL) Student Planner
Grade 9
ISBN: 978-1-7336417-8-4

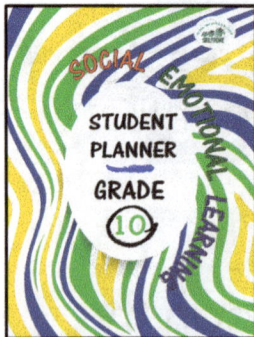

Social Emotional Learning
(SEL) Student Planner
Grade 10
ISBN: 978-1-7336417-9-1

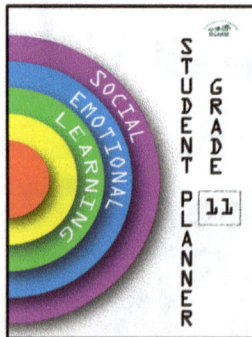

Social Emotional Learning
(SEL) Student Planner
Grade 11
ISBN: 978-1-7336417-4-6

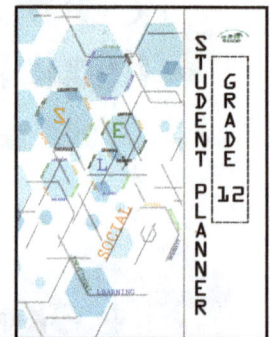

Social Emotional Learning
(SEL) Student Planner
Grade 12
ISBN: 978-1-7336417-5-3

For further information go to www.seltrove.com